1 0 1   W A Y S

TO IMPROVE YOUR PHARMACY WORKLIFE

1 0 1 WAYS
TO IMPROVE YOUR PHARMACY WORKLIFE

Mark R. Jacobs, R.Ph.

American Pharmaceutical Association
Washington, D.C.

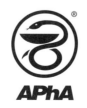

APhA

Acquiring Editor: Robert J. Howard
Editor: Vicki Meade, Meade Communications
Layout and Graphics: Cynthia Tourison, Modified Concepts
Cover Design: Mary Jane Hickey
Illustrator: John Moss, Moss Design
Proofreader: Mary De Angelo, Inkwell Communications
Indexing: Mary Coe

© 2001 by the American Pharmaceutical Association
Published by the American Pharmaceutical Association
2215 Constitution Avenue, N.W.
Washington, DC 20037-2985
www.aphanet.org
All rights reserved

No part of this book may be reproduced, stored in a retrieval system, or transmitted in any form or by any means, electronic, mechanical, photocopying, recording, or otherwise, without written permission from the publisher. The publisher makes no representation, express or implied, with regard to the accuracy of the information contained in this book and cannot accept any legal responsibility or liability for any errors or omissions that may be made.

To comment on this book via e-mail, send your message to the publisher at aphabooks@mail.aphanet.org

Library of Congress Cataloging-in-Publication Data

Jacobs, Mark R., R.Ph.
    101 ways to improve your pharmacy worklife / Mark R. Jacobs.
    p. cm.
    ISBN 1-58212-014-5
    1. Pharmacy—Practice. 2. Pharmacists. 3. Stress management. I. Title: One hundred one ways to improve your pharmacy worklife.

RS122.5 .J33 2000
615'.1'068—dc21   00-048090

How to Order This Book
By phone: 800-878-0729
(802-862-0095 from outside the United States)
VISA®, MasterCard®, and American Express® cards accepted.

DEDICATION

To my pharmacist wife, Brenda,
and our two daughters,
Ashley and Jessica.

CONTENTS

LIST OF IDEAS

Chapter 1 Changing the Way We Work

Chapter 2 Communication

Chapter 3 Employee Roles

Chapter 4 Tips for Managers and Supervisors

Chapter 5 Taking Control of Your Work Day

Chapter 6 The New Art of Delegating

Chapter 7 Workflow

Chapter 8 Third Party Issues

Chapter 9 The Telephone and Cash Register

Chapter 10 Doctors and Nurses

Chapter 11 Managing Your Time with
Pharmaceutical Representatives

Chapter 12 Professionalism

ACKNOWLEDGEMENTS

This book would not have been possible without the support and help of many people. To my former supervisor, Ken Schaefer, thank you for your never-ending encouragement and your belief that anything is possible. You have instilled in me Nike's "Just Do It" attitude and you've shown me how to get more out of the profession by focusing on what has value rather than what is merely urgent. I salute you for lifting me up when I've fallen and for helping me to truly think "outside of the box" rather than try to cram more into it.

I also thank Jerry Sveum, a friend and mentor who has encouraged my involvement in the profession on both a state and national level. A model communicator, Jerry has always had an optimistic outlook for the profession and has supported the vision of pharmaceutical care. Because he invited me to a semiprivate function at the 1994 American Pharmaceutical Association (APhA) meeting, I saw Jeanne Ann Stasny's model for a program called "Pharm Care"—a program that helped set the wheels in motion for widespread, positive changes in the profession.

Jeanne Ann's work inspired me and showed me what pharmaceutical care might look like. I and the profession are eternally indebted to her.

Thanks to the Pharmacy Society of Wisconsin for allowing me to contribute my talents, and for helping me develop into a better pharmacist. I would like to thank Chris Decker, Scott Whitmore, John Benske, Sue Kleppin, Chad Nechval, and the entire staff for all their behind-the-scenes work.

At APhA, I would like to thank April Shaughnessy for her support when I was a relatively new practitioner and for her groundwork with the Strategic Tactical Analysis Team Committee on Quality of Work Life. Thanks also to Jann Skelton, Lucinda Maine, Anne Burns, Susan Winckler, and to the committee's current staff liaisons for working to address problems near and dear to a lot of pharmacists.

To my staff of seven years—Sue Evans, Jane Yeager, Linda Blum, Deb Bentz, Shirley Hiatt, Linda Noss, and Don Dittmar—thank you for sticking it out with me. You have supported some crazy notions, often taking them and making them even better. You are the best pharmacy team anyone could ask for and deserve tremendous credit for improving the level of care that we are able to provide to our patients. And thank you to former staff pharmacist Chris Klink for the time he spent with us. Your vision and sales skills were instrumental in establishing appointments with patients and in achieving reimbursement.

Finally, and most importantly, I thank my pharmacist wife and friend, Brenda Jacobs, for listening to me talk pharmacy 16 hours a day and for supporting my constant and sometimes frustrating drive to improve the pharmacy work environment. She has successfully incorporated patient care into her practice and has received letters from doctors praising her for her ability to help their patients. She and Deana Leavens, a pharmacist with whom Brenda used to practice, have always impressed me with their service to patients and their ability to obtain reimbursement from insurance companies that is commensurate with the value of their work.

I also thank Brenda for being such a great mom to our lovely daughters, Jessica and Ashley. I love you all.

INTRODUCTION

Making time to incorporate new patient services into a pharmacy setting is tremendously challenging. When changes are proposed by managers or even by peers, pharmacists commonly say things like "we can't do that," "that won't work," or "not in my area." But today, changes are inevitable as pharmacists attack problems related to the explosion of new drugs in the marketplace, the aging population, and the restrictions of managed care. The demands on pharmacists will only get worse and erode our morale further if we don't take steps now to reshape our work environment—making it more professionally rewarding and better attuned to patients' health care needs.

This book describes real-life strategies for enhancing professionalism, improving job satisfaction, and reducing stress. The first 11 chapters provide concrete suggestions about time management, prioritizing, and communication, while Chapter 12 focuses on enhanced professionalism and a stronger patient care emphasis.

These approaches have been tried and proven effective in the busy chain pharmacy where, for eight years, I've been the pharmacy manager. Like you, I work in the trenches and I actively seek solutions to problems in our changing work environment. The 101 ideas this book puts forth are not "ivory tower" approaches or idealistic notions developed by academics or association managers who don't know what it's really like in the workplace.

Believe me, over the years I've been stressed out, overwhelmed, yelled at, and generally dissatisfied. Like most busy pharmacists, I tried to do everything for everyone while juggling technical duties, phone calls to physicians, and constant interruptions. I can relate to the way practitioners struggle in their current work environment and to their desire for a more professional atmosphere.

In 1994, when I attended the American Pharmaceutical Association's annual meeting in Seattle, Washington, my enthusiasm for pharmacy practice was reignited and I came away with a strong desire to provide a higher level of care to my patients than I had been. Among the speakers I listened to was Jeanne Ann Stasny, a pharmacist who described her cutting-edge program for implementing disease state management in a retail pharmacy. "Pharmaceutical care" was the buzzword that year, and hearing everyone talk about it motivated me to pursue my passion for helping people. I couldn't wait to get home and try some of the ideas I had acquired.

My first task though, was to share what I had learned by giving a presentation to pharmacy managers in another district in the large company where I work. I was enthusiastic and felt I presented a convincing case for why the profession must move towards enhanced patient care. I believed that pharmacists would welcome the ideas I shared with a sigh of relief, and that they would be quick to adopt this new practice model.

It was just the opposite. In response to my presentation I heard the three objections I referred to earlier in this introduction. It was as if the pharmacists were saying, "That might work in other parts of the country, but you don't know my customers!"

Determined to make patient care a reality, I decided I would try *anything* to improve my work environment. Working as a team with pharmacists and technicians in my pharmacy, we developed a plan. Not all the pharmacists and technicians originally bought into this plan, but when they started seeing the results—such as reduced stress, smoother operations, and better patient care—they began supporting the approaches. They even offered suggestions to make them more successful. Eventually I compiled the best ideas into this book.

Increased Satisfaction—Our Responsibility

An important outcome of the changes in our pharmacy is increased feelings of satisfaction and professionalism. Editorials and reports in national pharmacy journals have documented time and again the nationwide problem with job dissatisfaction among pharmacists today. A 1999 survey of 2000 pharmacists by Patrick McHugh, assistant professor of human resources management and labor relations at George Washington University, revealed that "more than 95% of respondents reported interruptions while filling a prescription order as a barrier to counseling patients." McHugh, whose study was designed to assess quality of worklife issues and identify crucial barriers to providing superior services, also discovered that "more than 90% of chains/supermarkets and independents said patient care is diminished, at least sometimes, because of time spent on insurance-related problems." Constant interruptions and time spent solving problems that shouldn't be pharmacists' responsibility lead to high levels of frustration.

In one of his columns in the newsletter of the National Association of Boards of Pharmacy, David Brushwood commented that many pharmacists believe "these are very, very bad times" because of the high stress of working in pharmacies. Brushwood, an attorney and professor of pharmacy health care administration at the University of Florida College of Pharmacy in Gainesville, goes on to say that pharmacists blame others for their plight: impatient patients, arrogant physicians, unsympathetic pharmacy supervisors, and even the boards of pharmacy. But pharmacists are at least partially responsible for their own problems, he points out, and are fully responsible for finding solutions—a viewpoint with which I heartily agree. It is up to pharmacists to make their work more professional and satisfying. No one is going to come in and do it for us.

Countless articles in pharmacy journals, magazines, and newsletters have focused on pharmaceutical care, disease state management, appointment-based practices, and reimbursement, but few of them have addressed the issue of the unprofessional work environments that so many pharmacists practice in. The articles tend to sound idealistic. In an editorial in the December 1996 issue of the *Journal of the American Pharmaceutical Association*, pharmacist Michael Webb said that ivory tower optimists "make repeated exhortations that the time for excuses is over and it is time we just do pharmaceutical care. I agree. My only question is, when? At what point in my day, filling 250 prescriptions in 12 hours, can I perform pharmaceutical care?"

Dealing with What's Important

This book was written for pharmacists seeking ideas for fitting pharmaceutical care into their busy days. In essence, it's a reference to help you bring about change. To my knowledge, no other book is available to help pharmacists make step-by-step alterations in their work environment. There are plenty of books and articles on pharmaceutical care, but few give you real-life examples of how to make time for it and get started.

While researching this book I found lots of general time management material, but it only teaches you how to work harder and faster to get more done. A more responsible approach, I believe, echoes the philosophy of Stephen Covey, leadership trainer and author of *The Seven Habits of Highly Effective People*. His principle of "first things first" focuses on accomplishing the *right* things and empowers you to achieve peace, balance, and fulfillment. He emphasizes that people should "deal with what's really important rather than responding to what's merely urgent."

Chapter 6 in this book, "The New Art of Delegating," can help you focus on what's really important—and relieve you of tasks that fill your time needlessly. With the time you free up you can concentrate on professional activities and get to the heart of problems that cost this country $76.6 billion a year—a figure that comes from a study led by J. Lyle Bootman, dean of the University of Arizona College of Pharmacy. The study, published in the *Archives of Internal Medicine* in 1995, indicated that illness and death associated with drug-related problems are more widespread than society had imagined. Many of these problems could be avoided, Bootman's study suggests, thus saving lives and reducing expenses for hospitalization, physician care, and emergency room visits.

In the book *Raving Fans*, Ken Blanchard—author of the famous *One Minute Manager*—offers three suggestions to create a "vision of perfection"centered around the customer. His suggestions provide a mental framework for making changes:

- **Decide what you want.** What would the perfect pharmacy look like? That is, how would the perfect pharmacy operate and be organized, and what would your role be in it?

- **Discover what the customer wants.** Looking after people's every whim doesn't work; often what they really want doesn't show up directly in what they say. "People who create raving fans as customers have minds of their own—no one can accuse them of being timid followers," Blanchard says. Are you a timid follower, or are you a leader?

- **Deliver plus one.** That is, deliver more than the customer ever imagined.

In today's fast-paced world there's just not enough time to "do it all." That's why this book is arranged into a series of 101 tips. You can quickly grasp one or two concepts and, in most cases, put them into effect in a very short time. Start with the easiest ones and be persistent in your efforts to make changes that will ultimately benefit patients. Change is very difficult for some people, so be kind to your coworkers as they struggle to adapt. But be tough on the issues you want to change.

There is no guarantee that, after implementing several or all of the strategies in this book, you will be able to do pharmaceutical care. However, I guarantee that if you incorporate some of these strategies you will at least reduce stress and gain control over your work environment. It's an opportunity to put some professionalism back into the profession.

A friend of mine suggested that I share something about the level of service we provide at our pharmacy. "Otherwise," he said, "your readers may not think that some of what you do will result in good service." Our company measures the service we provide by hiring an outside consulting firm to conduct telephone surveys with our customers. Recently we exceeded the corporate average on all 16 parameters the surveyors focus on, including whether customers received their prescriptions when promised, found the atmosphere professional, trusted the pharmacy, and felt the pharmacist was accessible when they wanted advice. For our success, I thank our entire pharmacy team, which worked together closely to shape and implement this book's methods.

I have made it my mission to help change the way we practice pharmacy. My strategies come from pharmacists like you, whose ideas I've borrowed and adapted after learning about them at association meetings and conferences. The term "pharmaceutical care" has been around for about 10 years now. Yet few have been able to actually do it, especially in large pharmacy chains. Let's get started.

CHAPTER 1

"We cannot solve

the problems of today with the

same thinking that got us here."

—Albert Einstein

Changing the Way We Work

Change is an essential part of any kind of growth. Yet people resist change. They find it uncomfortable to leave behind old ways of doing things and adopt new behaviors. This chapter gets you thinking about change and integrates ideas to help you make your first steps. To prepare for change, people need to begin with an open mind about it. Our perception of and willingness to accept change can mean the difference between success and failure.

 Idea #1 Become a change advocate.

Because change is so critical, it's the first topic I'm addressing in this book. Think about how often you hear the phrases "paradigm shift" and "thinking outside of the box." Both of these expressions, standard jargon among successful business people, have to do with change. To achieve your ambitions you must be willing to look at things differently. Change must be embraced with passion. When you master the art of change, you find that you can master just about anything.

In the box on the next page is a 10-step plan for change. Fill in the blanks and see how your answers match up with the actions that are fundamental to each step.

10-Step Plan For Change

1) _____ what you want to change.

2) Develop a _____ for change and decide to never go back.

3) Share your plan with your staff.

4) Elicit their _____.

5) Take a positive approach. Identify all the negative effects ahead of time. Then ask, "How can we make this work?"

6) _____ that there could be small failures along the way.

7) Remember, most people who succeed fail more than anyone else.

8) _____ your plan.

9) Notice whether your plan is working. And . . .

10) Make any necessary changes.

Answers: 1) Decide 2) Plan 4) Support 6) Accept 8) Implement

When John D. Rockefeller was asked for his prediction of the stock market he replied, "One thing is for certain, it will always change."

"Be willing to accept a temporary inconvenience for a permanent improvement." —H. Jackson Brown, Jr.

Idea #2 *Implement change immediately.*

SEE
RELATED
IDEA
#4

When you learn about a new idea, just do it! As I've already suggested, change is often disregarded because it's not within our comfort zone. My advice: If you hear about new strategies for success that sound good, implement them immediately.

Have you ever gone to a seminar or program where they were giving information that you thought was the greatest thing since the invention of string cheese, and you knew it was something that would really be of benefit? But then, instead of acting on the information, you put it aside because, gosh, you had to clean the house, or mow the lawn . . . or fill prescriptions and do inventory?

One of the most successful strategies I have learned is this: When I attend a state or national association meeting, I take away one or two great ideas we can implement immediately in our pharmacy.

Many people worry that they must work out all the details first. They think, "We'll have to get this all down on paper, then we'll have to review it with management, and then we'll have to have a meeting, or two, or three." They discuss it repeatedly, and then maybe it gets tabled because "We gotta figure out how we're going to enter this new insurance plan in the computer. And, oh well, it probably wouldn't have worked anyway."

Just do it! Accelerate the process of change in your work environment.

You know the saying, "If you always do what you always did, then you will always get what you always got"? My version of it goes like this:

"If you always do what you always did . . . then you will ALWAYS do what you have always done."

It sounds redundant doesn't it? But if you think about it awhile, it makes sense. If you don't start somewhere to do things differently, you will never do things differently. And, as the original saying suggests, you will never get different results.

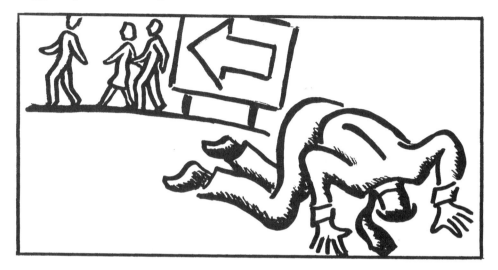

The next time some of your staff resist change, ask the nonbelievers to "just try it" for 21 days. Then they can go back to the old way of doing things if they want. It has been said that it takes 21 days to change a habit. You might be surprised at what becomes of your idea. Some people will continue to resist, but others will take it and make it better. It's okay if your idea ends up looking different than it did when you first introduced it. The important thing is that you moved forward with it.

Idea #3 Set a standard pickup time for special orders.

Here's an idea for your first small change. During the day, many pharmacies run short of an item or receive a request for something they don't stock. So they have to order it. For years our orders would arrive the next day at 11:00 am, plus or minus an hour. When patients would ask what time to come back for their medication, everyone had a different reply. "Oh, sometime around 10:30 or 11:00," we would generally say, wanting to give the fastest service possible.

The next day, the patient would come in for the medication. Sometimes it was ready, sometimes it was in the shipping tote, and sometimes it hadn't arrived yet. If the patient wasn't a little irritated or upset the day before, he most certainly felt inconvenienced now.

A couple years ago, when we discussed this issue at a staff meeting, we realized that by attempting to give excellent service, we were in fact giving poor service. "If we set a realistic expectation of when next-day orders will be ready instead of focusing on when they will arrive," a technician said, "then we can provide good service to all." We decided to set 2:00 pm as the time after which patients could arrive to pick up orders, allowing us plenty of flexibility to put the order away and fill leftover prescriptions from the previous day.

This simple change in the way we communicated to our patients resulted in increased customer satisfaction. Furthermore, delaying the pickup hour gave us extra time to call patients before they arrived if there was a problem with their order.

"Nothing is particularly hard if you divide it into small jobs." —Henry Ford

 Idea #4 Prepare everyone for change.

Because people become uneasy and uncertain when they move outside their comfort zone, the first step to making a change is to prepare for it.

This is especially important for larger changes that require everyone to work cohesively. A good way to pave the way for major changes—new approaches to carrying out key pharmacy operations, for example—is to hold a meeting where you ask questions to start a dialogue:

- "Tell me about a time when something changed in your life."
- "How did that make you feel?"

- "In time, did you find that the new way of doing things improved upon the old way?" (If no, ask, "Can you think of something that changed for the better?")

You might lead the direction of the discussion into pharmacy, if it is not already there, by asking, "Does anyone remember how difficult it was when we changed computer systems?" You could also ask, "Does anyone remember how the old computer system worked?" After some discussion, summarize the point you're making: "We found that our new computer system was difficult and challenging at first, but soon it became a better way of doing things."

Once your staff is comfortable talking about change, it's time to solicit their ideas. Find out what is really frustrating about each person's job. Let them know that you are gathering information, and that you will enlist their support for making positive changes. Emphasize that changes will be made "one thing at a time," rather than all at once. (You want to prepare them for incremental changes so they don't get impatient and think, "Nothing ever changes around here.") Be sure to remind them that changes might be uncomfortable at first, but that the long-term benefits are likely to outlive any short-term difficulties. If you sense resistance, you can say something like: "If after three to four weeks the majority of the staff still does not like the change, we can always go back."

"Any change, even a change for the better, is always accompanied by drawbacks and discomforts."

—Arnold Bennett

Idea #5 *Focus on what has value.*

SEE RELATED IDEA #42, 44, 46, 47

Details . . . details . . . So much to do, so little time. Too often, we get caught up in our day-to-day activities and forget what takes priority. In pharmacy, everything seems urgent!

Pharmacists and technicians can be like little wind-up toys. Just like in the commercial about Energizer batteries, we keep "going and going" until we run into a wall, and then we get stuck there. We do everything for everyone—and we do it *right now*. We probably devote no more than 15 seconds to any one task before an interruption occurs. Is it any wonder that working in a pharmacy is so stressful?

By doing so many things for so many people we are cheating the patient of our most valuable skills and ourselves of a career that should be professionally rewarding and enjoyable. The *Arthur Anderson Pharmacy Activity Cost and Productivity Study* appearing in *Drug Store News* in January 2000 found that pharmacists spend more than two-thirds of their work time on nonclinical and "nonjudgmental" tasks that "could be performed by nonpharmacists and/or be automated."

Automation can help free pharmacists' time, but it isn't the entire answer. Neither is delegating every nonprofessional task to technicians, who are limited by the number of functions they can handle. In many pharmacy work environments, when the technician workload is filled to capacity, pharmacists end up performing technical functions because no one else is available to do them. So consider which tasks you can eliminate entirely. Many successful people have accomplished great things by focusing on what has value and ignoring the small stuff.

In our pharmacy, putting the responsibility on patients to call their physicians for refills and iron out problems with their insurance providers frees up the pharmacists' time. Now we can make as many as two to three appointments per day with patients, provide disease state management for people with diabetes and asthma, and modify drug therapy with physician approval. Not only can we offer services at a higher professional level, but we can bill for our time, bringing in additional revenue.

To figure out what to change or eliminate, start by imagining the perfect work environment. In my perfect work environment I would spend most of my time on professional functions, including:

- patient consultation
- verifying prescriptions for safety and effectiveness
- drug utilization review
- one-on-one appointments with patients for disease state management
- health screening services

- administering immunizations
- co-managing patient drug therapy with physicians to improve clinical, humanistic, and economic outcomes

I am passionate about making this dream come true, and I will not give up until we get there. Now it's your turn—grab a pen and a notepad, and write down what your perfect work environment would be like.

My Perfect Work Environment

_____

_____

_____

_____

_____

_____

_____

_____

_____

_____

_____

_____

_____

Useful Ideas for Change Can Come from Unlikely Inspirations

After implementing many of the ideas in this book, we wanted to do more for our patients with the extra time we'd made available. One of our "value added" services—an idea that came to me in a flash of seemingly goofy inspiration—takes only a little extra effort on our part but is hugely appreciated by our patients. We call it "bunny service."

You're probably wondering, "What in the world is bunny service?" Basically, it's a program that restricts our speediest turnaround for filling prescriptions to patients who need it the most.

A few years ago one of our technicians, whose hobby is ceramics, brought in little brown bunnies about two inches high to give away as free gifts to any employee who wanted one. They sat on the counter for several days. No one was taking them. I took two and sat them on my desk. For weeks I stared at them wondering what to do with these bunnies. Then I came up with a plan.

Why not offer rapid service to patients who are feeling ill or have just been discharged from the hospital? In our next staff meeting, we talked about this idea. We decided that if patients requested fast service, or if we noticed they needed it, we would place a brown ceramic bunny in their prescription order basket (see idea #49) to signify that the prescription is high priority and must be filled in less than five minutes.

Our biggest concern was, what if everyone wants bunny service? It was a chance we had to take. If everyone asked for bunny service, we'd have to cancel the program. We laughed and joked about how people might abuse the service, creating all kinds of negative possibilities in our minds. But we've been offering bunny service for more than two years now, and no one has abused it. And our patients are so grateful. Comments like, "Wow, that was fast!" and "I'm really glad you could do this for me," are common. Our simple "bunny service" concept has helped create loyal patients, a caring atmosphere, and a positive image for our pharmacy.

Here's the sign we use to promote this service.

ATTENTION

If you or a member of your family is feeling ill, please let us know and we will fill your prescription immediately for you.

Idea #6 Cross train all pharmacy staff.

Having a fully functional staff can make a big difference in daily stress levels. Each person has primary responsibilities and often staffers are hesitant to do anything other than their regular duties. But when the person with primary responsibility for a task is on break, sick, on vacation, or on their day off, someone has to fill in. Too often, that "someone" is the pharmacist.

Have all your team members write down their responsibilities. (Even if you only have two employees, there are benefits to cross training.) Now you have a list of most of the tasks in your department. From this list, you can identify who needs to be trained in which tasks so that everyone is cross trained.

As you undergo this exercise, think about delegating to others responsibilities that currently belong to the pharmacist. Some tasks historically done by pharmacists are now considered nonprofessional or technical in nature, and many are no longer required by law to be handled by a pharmacist. Some tasks that can be delegated include filling prescriptions, setting the staffing schedule, placing drug orders to wholesalers or manufacturers, and dealing with prescription returns. In most states, the only things a pharmacist must do are check the final prescription, consult with patients, and take prescriptions over the phone.

Initially, some pharmacists may worry that "technicians won't be able to do as good a job." That may be true for a few days, because everyone makes some mistakes when they learn a new task. But soon they will master the new duties. In our department, technicians do essentially everything that does not legally require a pharmacist, and quite honestly, they are as good or better.

CHAPTER 2

"When the mind expands

to incorporate a new idea,

it will never shrink to its original size."

—*Author unknown*

Communication

Idea #7 Train patients to call 24 hours in advance for refills.

With the right attitude and plenty of reinforcement, it's possible to get patients used to calling a day ahead of time for prescription refills. In our pharmacy, every time we receive a prescription refill request with less than two hours' notice—including those dropped off at the prescription window—we give the patient the letter below. We place it in the bag with each patient's prescriptions and we verbally reinforce it with every consultation.

There's no need to be negative. A good approach is to kindly explain, "We are now offering a new service we believe will allow us to help everyone faster. The next time you need a prescription refilled, if you would call it in a day ahead of time we will be able to provide better service to everyone. If you still need it that day, we will be happy to fill it for you."

Dear Patient,

We are now offering "no wait" prescription refill service. While we are happy to fill any of your prescriptions on a moment's notice, we ask that for refill prescriptions you give us 24 hours' notice, or even a few hours if you need the prescription the same day.

By calling in your prescription ahead of time, it allows us to serve you faster, and also to take care of patients who are feeling ill. By giving 24 hours' notice, you will be guaranteed "no wait" for your prescriptions.

We appreciate your business.

Thank you!

It's always a negotiation game. Some people will play, some will not. The change is slow, but if everyone on the pharmacy staff communicates consistently and positively, you will notice a considerable increase in the time you have available to help your patients. Since we implemented this effort, more than half (60% to 70%) of all our refill requests are for pickup later that day or the following day. This gives us extra time to provide consultation or fit in appointments for services such as diabetes education.

Patients will need help making this transition. In fact, one major chain pharmacy trains its technicians to ask the simple question, "When would you like to pick this up?" whenever a patient drops off a prescription. They are reconditioning the patient to choose a time other than "now." Below are other examples of ways to communicate effectively:

- **Verbal communication on a phone request, especially for three or more refills.** "Would you like that tomorrow, or later on today?" Notice that, in this example, "right away" or "in 20 minutes" were not even presented as choices. Give patients whatever they want, but keep conditioning them to recognize that "tomorrow" is a favorable option.

- **Verbal communication at the pickup window.** "Let me tell you about our 'no wait' prescription refill service. Did you know that if you call in your prescription 24 hours in advance, we guarantee that it will be ready and waiting when you arrive?"

Idea #8 Stamp receipts with a reminder to call
24 hours in advance.

Changing the patient's expectations takes time. A technique that has worked well for us is stamping all prescription receipts with red ink to say:

PLEASE CALL 24 HOURS
IN ADVANCE FOR FASTER
REFILL SERVICE.

Put this message on a simple rubber stamp. Use the stamp regularly and not only will patients become conditioned, but you will be on your way to a more efficient work environment.

Idea #9 Explain the benefits of your new "call ahead" service every chance you get.

If patients don't take advantage of calling in their refills in advance, neither party benefits. The benefit to the pharmacy is clear: Getting a day's notice on refills reduces the number of functions that require immediate attention. It takes pressure off the pharmacists. But what is the customer service angle? Patients always wants to know, "What's in it for me?" Your job is to tell them.

Even if your pharmacy uses an electronic interactive voice response system (IVR) for refills, it's important to continually explain your "call ahead" refill service. There are at least four opportunities to tell patients about your call ahead service and change their refill ordering habits:

1. Telephone Refills. When patients call for refills on the telephone, make a note on their refill receipt. A simple note, such as "explain CAR [call ahead refill] service," reminds the pharmacist that the patient's arrival to pick up the prescription will be an opportunity to explain the service to the patient. You've already made progress by training the patient to call in advance, but the call ahead service does little good if patients phone only to say they'll be right over. To start weaning patients from the idea that they can call and get prescriptions filled immediately, pick a set interval—such as 30 minutes—as the estimated time that the prescription will be ready. Then gradually increase the interval until you've established a standard time frame that is reasonable for both the pharmacy and the patients. In our pharmacy, as a general rule, we tell callers who want immediate service that their prescription will be ready in an hour.

When patients call for refills, tell them about the ability to call 24 hours in advance, as in idea #7, and follow this with, "If you forget to call in your refill a day ahead of time, you can also call in the morning or after work, or even a few hours ahead." If they ask, let them know that you are always willing to refill prescriptions on a moment's notice.

In response to the question in the patient's mind, "What's in it for me," you can explain that calling ahead allows you to make sure patients don't have to wait when they arrive at the pharmacy, and makes it possible for you to take better care of patients who feel sick and need immediate service. Simply telling patients that you can't put 30 pills in a bottle in 15 minutes will not convince them to call ahead, but most people can relate to not feeling well. Let your patients know that you also have a priority service set up (as described in idea #7) to help them when they are not feeling well and need their prescriptions immediately.

2. At Intake Window. Promote your call ahead refill service at the prescription intake window. It doesn't have to be a lengthy, earth-shattering conversation. Try this. "Hi, Mrs. Jones. How are you today? [Exchange niceties.] Did you know that you can call in your prescription refills a day ahead of time, or even a few hours in advance on the same day, and we'll have them ready for you when you get here?"

Good. Now practice saying it with a smile the whole time. Be sure to tell Mrs. Jones that her prescription will be ready in 10 to 15 minutes, or whatever is reasonable in your pharmacy.

3. In Pickup Area. A third opportunity for explaining your call ahead refill service is when patients are in the prescription pickup or consultation area. It's really no different from explaining the service at the prescription intake window. To communicate what's in it for the patient, you can call it your "no wait" prescription refill service. If patients don't understand your priority to help sick people first, they will most likely find value in a "no wait" prescription refill service.

4. When Apologizing. Probably my favorite opportunity for explaining the "no wait" refill service is when a customer has had the unfortunate experience of waiting too long for a refill. After you have apologized to the patient for the delay, you can introduce your "no wait" service this way, for example: "Mr. Conway, I apologize for the long wait today. You deserve better service than that. I would like to include a note about our "no wait" prescription refill service in your bag. Next time, if you would call in your prescription a few hours in advance, I assure you it will be ready for you when you arrive. Thank you for your patience, and have a great day."

Your tone should be apologetic and directed at being helpful. Remember, there is no excuse for patients receiving poor service that day. When patients are not receptive to your being helpful, then revert back to being apologetic. Express how much you appreciate their business and emphasize your desire to do a better job next time.

 Idea #10 Condition patients to ask doctors for new prescription orders when refills expire.

SEE RELATED IDEA #20, 42

Pharmacy work environments are fraught with problems and interruptions that keep us from helping people. How many pharmacists spend the first hour of their morning calling doctors regarding expired prescriptions for which patients sought refills at the pharmacy the day before? And throughout the day, they make many more such calls. The time pharmacists waste dealing with expired prescriptions is a major impediment to our ability to consult with patients and help them with their medication-related problems.

Good communication skills are the key to successfully dealing with patients who have expired refills. On a phone-in prescription refill request, what if you were to say to the patient:

- "Mrs. Jones, did you realize that the prescription you called in today is out of refills?"

- "Do you happen to have a new prescription from your doctor?"

- "Would you like me to give you a couple of tablets to hold you over until you are able to get hold of your doctor?"

I am constantly surprised at the responses I receive after returning calls to patients who have phoned in expired refills. When I use the lines above, often what I hear is:

- "Oh . . . I'm sorry, I didn't even realize it was expired. I'll call my doctor."
- "I've got a new prescription and I'll bring it in with me."
- "Okay, so what do I need to do?"
- "I'll get hold of my doctor for a new prescription."

Changing patients' habits regarding refills is a sensitive matter in most pharmacies. Coming across as rude or insensitive is the last thing you want to do. You can avoid this pitfall by having a canned response posted by each of the phones, as explained in idea #20. Making standard, printed responses available will help train your staff to communicate positively and ease the way toward effective change. Pharmacies that have stopped calling doctors for refills have told me that they've seen positive changes in their professional work environment and that they will not revert to their old ways.

If you open a constructive dialogue with patients about taking responsibility for their refills, the worst case scenario is that they resist taking action and you end up calling the doctor yourself. However, most of them will begin calling their own doctor for refills, leaving you more time to focus on basic patient consultation, disease state management, and pharmaceutical care.

For more details on this important concept, see idea #42. The important thing to remember is that how we communicate with patients is a powerful tool.

Idea #11 Cast yourself as a consultant.

Early in my career I felt as though no one respected me as a health care professional. Sure, we were the "most trusted" professionals for nine consecutive years, according to annual Gallup polls, but it seemed to me that respect wasn't always there.

After attending a seminar on communication, I began to ask myself if I was really doing all I could to communicate professionally and engender respect. I thought about how Lexus no longer sells "used" cars, they're "pre-owned." I wondered, how can we adapt this strategy to the pharmacy profession?

In our pharmacy, we used to discuss the high cost of medications with patients, then offer to *call* their doctor to *switch* to a *cheaper drug*. After I considered this message more carefully, I realized that the words in italics describe technical functions that, it seems, anyone could do. I began to do some word-smithing and came up with a different sentence: "Mrs. Jones, if you would like, I will *consult* with your physician, *discuss therapeutic alternatives*, and see if we can find *a medication that is equally or more effective at a lower cost.*"

See the difference a few changes can make? Not only did we change how we communicated our message, but we started to charge for it! By not giving away our information for free, we also communicated value. One patient paid us over $100 for saving him money on a therapeutic alternative.

So, make sure you are portraying a professional image when communicating to patients and that you are using terminology that emphasizes, rather than undermines, your knowledge.

 ## Idea #12 Intervene rather than override.

When a technician asks a pharmacist to do an *override* on the computer for an alert that pops up about a potential problem, is it considered a technical function or one requiring professional judgment? We discussed this in a staff meeting and decided it required professional judgment and therefore should be referred to as an *intervention*.

All day long, technicians would call out, "I need an *override*, I need an *override*." It sounded so technical. "Override" means to set aside or bypass an automatic function. When we talk about "interventions," we're referring to acts that require professional judgment and are done on behalf of a patient's well-being. Which do you prefer to hear?

Idea #13 Change from "customer" to "patient."

Do you refer to your clients as *customers* or as *patients*? Although we know our clients are customers, they are also people receiving health care—which means they are patients. We wanted to make a switch in vocabulary, but didn't want it to take five or six weeks like "intervention" did.

We knew from experience that it's difficult for one or two pharmacists to monitor and correct communication, so we enlisted the support of the entire staff. If they monitored each other, we thought, it would also be more effective than if the pharmacists were the "bad guys" all the time. To make it fun, we brought in a bowl of hard candies and instituted this game: Every time a technician said the word customer, the first staffer to point out the communication error got a piece of candy. To add extra impact, the person making the error had to go over to the bowl and get the candy for the person who'd caught them. You can imagine how humiliating this could be if it happened regularly. Within two weeks the problem was corrected, and there was still candy left in the bowl.

We used to overhear technicians say to callers who wanted to reach the pharmacist, "He's talking to a customer." It makes us feel good about our jobs to hear what technicians say now: "The pharmacist is *consulting* with a *patient* on his *medication therapy* at the moment. Would you like to hold?"

Idea #14 Display your credentials.

You've probably heard it said that "perception is reality." Well, the public's perception of what we do is their reality. Some people still believe that pharmacists go to school to learn how to read doctors' handwriting and count by fives. One person was surprised when I informed him that I went to school for six years and then did a one-year internship. He thought that maybe pharmacy required only a two-year degree. Sound familiar?

SEE RELATED IDEA #48, 93

If pharmacists ever expect to get paid for anything other than dispensing, changing public perception is critical.

What's the first thing you see when you enter a doctor's office? Usually some degrees framed on the wall, as well as certificates for fellowship training, residencies, board certification, specialties, and the like. These visible credentials build confidence that the person you are seeing has expertise in a given area of medicine.

Post your pharmacy degree, plaques for serving as an instructor or preceptor, pharmacy association awards, board certification documents, and certificates for disease state management training. The state of Wisconsin has a professional-looking document available from the board of pharmacy with the governor's signature on it—perhaps your state has the same.

Hang as many of these items on the wall as you can without creating clutter. (If several pharmacists' credentials are to be displayed, it's probably wise to have a limit of three or four certificates per person.) Once patients see that you are certified and licensed in a multitude of areas, chances are you will gain additional respect.

 **Idea #15 Wear a clean smock every day.
Or don't wear one at all!**

I've often mentioned to colleagues that I think we should stop wearing smocks. Whoa! This one hits a nerve with some pharmacists. But think about it: How you dress is a form of nonverbal communication. Image is everything. Some reasons to consider removing your smock:

- Smocks are antiquated and associated with the past.
- Many physicians don't wear white jackets anymore, and nurses have lost those funny-looking hats.
- It's not necessary for all health care professionals to look alike. Professional skill and demeanor are what matter, not the specific outfit we wear.

Smocks do nothing to change our image from pill dispenser to health care professional. People tend to associate our smocks with drug products. Let's turn the public's attention to the pharmacist as the expert in the area of medication knowledge and services, rather than the vendor of pills. Removing the smock is a great way to say, "We really care about you, and our focus is now on you, not just the drug." As you make changes in your pharmacy services and operations, removing your smock is a highly visible sign that things are different now.

Some pharmacists, however, like wearing a smock, and some are required to wear them by their employers. I've heard pharmacists argue that smocks help establish a consistent image in the public's mind and also help patients quickly identify which staff person is the pharmacist. Others contend that smocks provide a place to put your name badge without leaving pin holes in nice clothes. In deciding for or against smocks, take into consideration how physicians and other health professionals dress in your area.

Do Smocks Make the Pharmacist?

Some pharmacists are concerned that they won't be recognized as pharmacists without their smocks. That's silly. When you talk to a doctor who's not wearing a white coat, do you worry that he or she isn't really a doctor? One female pharmacist strongly objected to my suggestion of removing her smock because she believed that garment was what made her recognizable to people as the pharmacist. I didn't have a good response at the time, but later that day, when I related the conversation to my wife—also a pharmacist—she told me this story. In a pharmacy where she used to work with four male pharmacists, patients did not acknowledge her as a pharmacist at first, even though they all wore smocks. But as soon as they realized how much she knew about medication therapy, they began looking to her for help. It was her knowledge and professional manner that brought about the shift, not her clothing.

If a smock is part of your professional attire, make sure you wear a clean one every day. When patients see us wearing dirty clothes it affects their perception of our profession and has an impact on the way they treat us.

What you wear underneath your smock is just as important. I once saw a pharmacist wearing an older, barber-style smock. It was not pressed, and to make matters worse, he was wearing a T-shirt under it. I don't think the way he presented himself did anything to help change the image of pharmacists from pill dispensers to care givers. And his clothing simply didn't look clean or professional. When smocks are worn, they should be crisp, fresh, and modern, with professional-looking garb beneath. Some pharmacists have their name and title monogrammed onto their smocks. That's a good idea; I applaud anything you can do to enhance your patients' perception of you.

Idea #16 Become a smile communicator.

What we say and how we say it can make a big difference in how we are perceived. Have you ever patted a dog on the head, smiled, and in a soft, polite tone told him that he was a bad dog for doing his business on the carpet? Chances are, he wagged his tail and thought, "Oh boy, my owner sure does like me!"

Don't misunderstand . . . I'm not comparing people to dogs. My point is that smiling and speaking in a soft, friendly tone can make a difference in how your words are received.

Smiling works on the telephone too; it comes through in your voice.

Components of Communication

7% = Words

38% = Tone of Voice

55% = Visual Cues

People tend to think of "communication" as the words we use, but words only convey a fraction of our meaning. Tone of voice, gestures, body language, and other nonverbal components make up the rest of the message.

Pharmacists and technicians are forced to communicate negative information on a regular basis. "Your refills are expired." "Your insurance company rejected your prescription." "You no longer have insurance coverage." "Your prescription is not ready yet."

This book gives many examples of effective ways to convey negative information to people. Whenever you speak to patients, add a sincere smile. Your smile shows genuine concern and can help reduce patients' stress.

Idea #17 The customer is **not** *always right.*

There are at least five situations in which the customer is not always right:

SEE RELATED IDEA #56, 57, 58

- When a customer's request runs counter to pharmacy laws.
- When the customer uses profanity.
- When sexual harassment is involved.
- When customers claim to be "shorted" on controlled substances and want the balance.
- When customers insist that you bill their insurance when an item is not covered or when their insurance has been terminated.

Certainly, this list is not all-inclusive. Other situations will inevitably come up. When Corporate America told us that "The customer is always right," I don't think they intended to say there are no exceptions. Pharmacists and technicians endure a great deal of stress as a result of taking this statement literally.

Perhaps the saying should be, "Make customers feel as if they are right, and respect their disappointment when things don't go exactly as they expected." But then that wouldn't be as catchy, would it?

When customers use profanity or sexually harass the pharmacy staff, it simply is *not acceptable.* No one should be under the impression that their employer expects them to endure these kinds of abuse. Any customer who exhibits such behavior should be asked to leave. And, depending on the severity of the offense, you should decide whether that customer will ever be allowed into your pharmacy again.

Some other situations in which the customer is not right—especially those related to pharmacy laws—are less cut and dried. When pharmacy laws create challenges, it is appropriate to do everything within the law to ensure that the patient receives the necessary medication. While we have a responsibility to ourselves and our profession, we also have an obligation to help people. If we do not care for the patients who come into our pharmacies, there is no future for "pharmaceutical care."

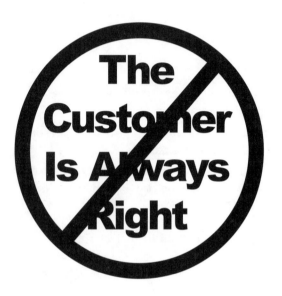

Patients' claims about being shorted on their medications are challenging to handle. Doing what's right takes judgment. It's one thing for patients to insist they didn't receive the correct amount of an antibiotic; it's another when they claim they were shorted on controlled substances. If the pharmacy staff cannot verify that the patient was, in fact, shorted by a specific amount, then other options must be considered, such as contacting the patient's physician. Has the patient made such claims before? Will he or she accept a refund? After resolving the issue with the patient, it never hurts to document in the patient's profile that his or her medication must be double counted. In our pharmacy, when patients have "double count" noted in their profile, we circle the quantity on the prescription label after double counting it and we initial the spot on the prescription stub where the words "double count" are printed.

Avoid the 'Drug Police' Mentality

I've seen situations in which pharmacists and technicians seem to think their primary role is to be "drug police." They can't wait to exercise their authority. I'd hate to see what would happen if they were given a pair of handcuffs! For example, I heard about a pharmacist who refused to fill a prescription for Duragesic patches because the physician had ordered more than the 30 days' supply allowed by state law. This prescription had been brought in by the relative of a known cancer patient. Instead of simply providing a month's worth of the medication and explaining that a new prescription order would be required for more, the pharmacist returned the prescription order to the relative and said, "Sorry, I can't fill this," without offering an explanation. The physician had probably made a simple mistake, which the pharmacist could have corrected with a quick phone call—thus providing excellent service to an extremely ill patient.

As for the last item on the list on page 25, dealing with third party issues takes communication skills that you can develop with practice. Ideas for handling these types of situations are discussed in Chapter 8: Third Party Issues.

Idea #18 Use "Here's what we can do" to diffuse anger or create a positive spin.

Nobody wants to hear bad news. Bad news can be a catalyst for a whole cascade of negative emotions. It can lead to a hostile dialogue, and nobody walks away happy. Place a pharmacist or technician in the position of having to deliver bad news on a regular basis and you have an instant recipe for stress, anxiety, and decreased job satisfaction.

When you have to give patients bad news, such as their medication isn't in stock or the price of a drug they need has gone up, the first step is to separate yourself emotionally from the problem. Next, focus on what you can do to make things right.

When I was a bagger at a grocery store in high school, a little old lady looked at me as I was bagging her groceries and said, "The last time I was here you squished my bread!" I don't think I was the person who actually did the squishing, but because her most recent bread purchase had been made at that store, she pegged me as the culprit. I told her I was sorry that her bread had gotten squished and explained that I was going to put it in the bag last so it wouldn't happen again. I did not become defensive or take her accusation personally—instead I diffused her anger by politely explaining how I would make things right this time.

Here, in more detail, are the two steps you should follow to handle situations involving bad news:

1. Keep emotional distance to avoid taking the problem personally. If you spend oodles of time working on one person's problem, and then are criticized for not solving it, the situation is more difficult for you now because you have taken ownership. You have also invested your time, which is limited to begin with. Instead of considering yourself personally responsible for the problem—the one who must handle all the details involved in solving it—imagine you are a consultant who coaches the patient about options for resolving the matter.

2. Recast the situation in a positive light by explaining the choices the patient has. This enlists the patient's help as part of a problem-solving team, with you as his ally. Joining forces with the patient to solve the problem allows the patient to separate the problem from *you*. Present the choices immediately, so the patient doesn't have as much time to think about the negative aspects of the situation. For example, if a patient's insurance refuses to pay for a prescription, "here's what we can do" could be offering to provide one or two days' worth of medication to allow the patient time to contact his or her employee benefits department. Then, as a second option, suggest that the patient pay cash now and let you know when the insurance problem is cleared up so you can resubmit the claim for a refund.

Also keep in mind visual communication strategies that can reinforce your position as an ally. When you stand across from the patient separated by a counter top, you have a visual barrier between you. This face-to-face position contributes to the patient's perception that it's a confrontation. To eliminate the visual barrier, use a "distracter," such as the person's prescription bottle, a rejection slip, or something else you can focus on together. Place the distracter to the left or right in such a way that it allows you to turn and face the same direction as the patient.

When possible, come out from behind the counter and stand side by side. It positions you to work together toward a mutually agreeable solution. And it's much more difficult for people to become angry with you when they can't look directly at your face. Some pharmacists add a personal touch by going out and sitting down next to the patient.

Practice Makes Perfect

Try this exercise to help improve your skills. Think of a situation you encountered in which you had to communicate bad news. Consider alternative ways to approach the same situation. Write a response using the "Here's what we can do" approach, and give the patient at least two choices. Now practice the scenario several times—role playing it with your staff—so the next time you are more comfortable handling it.

Idea #19 Use humor daily.

Humor is important in any work environment. Pharmacies are so busy, it can seem difficult to find time for humor, and you may worry about the image you're conveying to patients standing nearby. Using humor the right way, however, can increase morale and job satisfaction. It can also reduce stress and improve relations with both employees and patients.

Be careful to avoid inappropriate humor—any joke or statement that pokes fun at a person or a group of people. Jokes that involve sex, religion, or politics are also good to steer away from, since people tend to have strong opinions on these topics. Humor that works best is directed at oneself or one's environment. It can also be used in response to a rhetorical question.

For example, patients often make sarcastic comments about the high cost of their medications. You might respond by joking that they should receive stock in the company. You might even add, "How many shares of stock would you like?"

Another opportunity for levity is when a patient comes to the prescription pickup window inquiring if the prescription dropped off earlier is ready yet. You could respond, "Oh yes . . . we had that ready *hours* ago," a ludicrous statement since it's been an hour or less since you received the prescription order. If the patient is in a good mood, you could continue by telling her that she is your best customer, or has been named "Customer of the Month." Most people enjoy a bit of banter or gentle teasing.

There are more than 50 different muscles in the face. When people exercise them by smiling, "feel good" neurotransmitters such as serotonin are released. These endogenous chemicals have a relaxing and calming effect on us.

Have fun with your staff, too. When they're least expecting it, make a comment such as, "I just want you all to know that you're the best group of technicians in this whole town. In fact, I would bet that you're the best group of technicians in the whole state!" Inevitably, someone will comment that it's getting thick in here, or that they're sorry they forgot their boots today.

Sometimes we ask the staff how many prescriptions they think are waiting to be picked up at a specific time. We kid around with them, saying that anyone who gets the number exactly right will be allowed to go home early. Someone usually responds with the question, "How early can we go home?" We tell them, "It depends on who gets it right!"

A couple of our technicians smoke. Occasionally I ask them if I can bum a cigarette off them. They find it funny because they know I don't smoke, and they know they have a bad habit that they should quit. When some of our staff asked me if I had any New Year's resolutions, I responded, "Yes, I've decided to take up smoking and I'm going to try to be a little meaner next year." They all chuckled.

Work should be fun. Most people spend 50% of their waking hours at work. Even if you haven't been enjoying yourself at work lately, adding a little humor can go a long way toward improving the atmosphere. Touches of lightheartedness will benefit everyone, and may help build the rapport necessary for effectively implementing changes in your work environment.

$\copyright$ H A P T E R 3

"Coming together is a beginning;

keeping together is progress;

working together is success."

—Henry Ford

Employee Roles

Idea #20 Post "canned responses" by each of the phones.

SEE RELATED IDEA #7, 10-14, 22, 26

What you say and how you say it can make a big difference as you implement changes in your pharmacy operations. It's important that everyone on staff communicates the same message to patients. But ensuring consistency among all staff can be a challenge. A short list of "canned" responses that you have planned in advance will help everyone in the department deliver a consistent message.

In idea #26, for example, we discuss obtaining four pieces of information from patients who phone in prescription refill requests: prescription number, first and last name, estimated time the patient will arrive to pick up the prescription, and phone number. The chances of having the entire staff remember which four items must be noted for every prescription refill request are marginal at best. Keeping a list near the telephone to jog the staff's memory is a huge help.

Another good time to use canned responses is when you are conditioning patients to call their doctors for refills when their prescriptions expire (idea #10). Post the items in the box on the next page next to your phone to remind staff of effective phrases.

Coaching Patients to Call Their Doctors for Refills

1. "Mrs. Jones, did you realize that the prescription you called in today is out of refills?"

2. "Do you happen to have a new prescription from your doctor?"

3. "Would you like me to give you a couple of tablets to hold you over until you are able to get hold of your physician?"

It's also very helpful to provide canned responses for technicians to use when you are busy helping another patient. For example: "The pharmacist is consulting with a patient right now. Would you like me to take your phone number and have her call you back?"

Consider placing canned responses on one quick reference sheet by each phone in the pharmacy department. Of course you don't need to copy verbatim the wording I've supplied. Take these ideas and modify them any way you see fit.

Idea #21 Provide technician mailboxes.

SEE RELATED IDEA #33

Giving each staff person a mailbox is a great way to share information about insurance company changes or other important matters. Health care policy is forever changing, and it has a major impact on the pharmacy environment. The sooner your entire staff has access to key information affecting your pharmacy, the more efficiently your operation will run.

If your staff already has mailboxes, don't let them be used only as cubbyholes for storing gum and name badges. Share important memos from the corporate office or relevant letters from insurance companies. If one insurance company is bought by another, for example, it's helpful for everyone to know as soon as possible.

You've all seen the bulk junk mail that comes to the pharmacy. Maybe it's not so junky. You can circulate some of it to staff to share information on new prescription drugs and over-the-counter products. Then the next time a patient asks about ordering a new product, or someone needs to interpret a medication order, your staff may already recognize the name and won't have to bother you. Routing some of your mail enhances your technicians' knowledge and makes your job easier in the process.

Of course, some of the information you receive is very technical. Because the staff doesn't need to know as much about each product as you do, it's a good idea to highlight or circle what you feel is important. Most of the time, the name of the product, the strength, and what it's used for will do. A simple way to forward the information is to attach a routing slip, as shown below.

**Place a checkmark next to your name
after you've looked at this; then pass it on.**

_____ Don

_____ Sue

_____ Linda

Circle one: Recycle or Return to: _____

Idea #22 *When a prescription is delayed, tell the patient as soon as possible.*

SEE
RELATED
IDEA
#20

Whenever a prescription is delayed, no matter what the reason, the patient should be informed as soon as possible. This is common sense. Even so, pharmacies may vary in how they handle delays, depending on who is on duty. A standard approach should be established and incorporated into your operating procedures.

If there are inconsistencies within your pharmacy, it may be beneficial to discuss the topic at a meeting. Start by asking your staff if situations ever arise in which a prescription is delayed. If possible, have an easel and a flip chart or paper to write on. Ask everyone to identify as many situations as possible that create delays.

After listing them all, start a new page and discuss ways to handle each instance. As your staff works through this exercise, informing the patient should emerge as top priority.

Patients you are trying to notify about delays can be in one of at least three places: in the pharmacy, in your store, or at home. If that's where they are, they're relatively easy to reach. But what do you do if the patient is calling from work or a cellular phone? Challenge the staff by presenting alternative scenarios. For example, one idea might be that you routinely obtain work phone numbers for future use. Another option would be to ask every patient calling in a refill to supply the phone number they are calling from. Based on this brainstorming exercise you can develop standard operating procedures for communicating delays. To ensure further consistency, you can also use idea #20 and have your pharmacy team write down canned responses to use when telling patients about delays.

When patients appear at the prescription window annoyed about a delay, we have found that we get a more favorable response if we tell them we will be working on their prescription next. (Or, if several people are waiting nearby, we might say, "There's only a couple of prescriptions ahead of yours, so it should be ready very soon.") If we were simply too busy to handle the workload—as opposed to delays caused by, say, the patient's insurance carrier—the last thing patients want to hear is, "It will be five to ten more minutes." Providing a specific amount of time sets you up to disappoint the patient. When a patient hears that he or she is "next," it eases some of the tension.

When your staff collaboratively agrees on the procedures, they will take ownership of them, and therefore will be more likely to follow through on them. Furthermore, this feeling of ownership will motivate them to monitor one another—so you don't have to.

Idea #23 Invite technicians to attend your local pharmacy meetings.

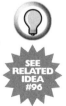

SEE RELATED IDEA #96

Technicians are the future of pharmacy. Like it or not, technology and supportive personnel will transform our profession as the population ages and we are hit with an increasing number of prescriptions. For pharmacists to be able to practice pharmacy, we need to include and educate technicians.

One way to do this is to start inviting them to local pharmacy meetings. After all, shouldn't technicians have access to the same networking opportunities that pharmacists do? At these gatherings, technicians can learn new ways to improve efficiency and free pharmacists' time to educate and consult with patients, monitor patient status, and follow up with physicians. At these meetings, include technicians in discussions that are relevant to the scope of their work, and urge them to voice their thoughts and concerns. Invite technicians to opening sessions, banquets, social events, and award ceremonies. And consider including a technician-only track for education geared to them specifically.

Doctors and nurses work together to improve patient care. Pharmacists and technicians can do the same. In fact, given the challenges in our current health care system, physicians, nurses, pharmacists, technicians, and other health professionals are likely to work more and more closely together to improve care, bridge gaps, and allow for a more seamless delivery of services. Integrating services and sharing knowledge will be key.

 Idea #24 Encourage technician certification.

Technicians are the backbone of any successful pharmacy operation. Often technicians become more proficient at certain tasks than the pharmacist. Educating technicians so that they can earn certification (which is awarded after successful performance on a standard exam), in addition to inviting them to pharmacists' meetings, will only serve to strengthen our profession.

Certifying technicians gives them credibility because they are measured by a universal standard, and it creates a unified pool of employees with a similar knowledge base. Of course there will be differences in knowledge and talents among individual technicians, but differences exist among people in any profession. Diversity has many plusses—but so does meeting a minimum standard of competency.

Forging a common bond among technicians and promoting their professional recognition through certification help create a "career" versus "job" mentality. It also can lead to increased job satisfaction. Technicians are likely to feel a sense of pride and dedication that goes with belonging to an elite group.

Encourage your technicians to take ownership in their profession by becoming certified. Contact your state pharmacy association for information on procedures and costs, or get in touch with the Pharmacy Technician Certification Board in Washington, D.C. (Telephone: 202-429-7576; website: www.ptcb.org). As an incentive to encourage their technicians to become certified, some pharmacies offer a pay increase of 50 cents per hour to those who pass the certification exam. Others provide financial assistance to offset the cost of the exam and study materials.

Idea #25 Don't duplicate effort — type information directly into the computer.

SEE RELATED IDEA #13

How many times each day does a new patient come to your prescription intake window, and the technician writes all the demographic and health history data directly on the paper prescription order? Then, when they have extra time (ha ha), they type the information into the computer. A good technician can, and should, enter new patient information directly into the computer. There is absolutely no reason why we should be doing the same task twice.

To help change your staff's behavior, use the "bowl of candy" approach explained in idea #13. When a technician is detected duplicating effort by typing patient information after first writing it longhand, he or she must go to the bowl and bring a piece of candy to whoever pointed out the duplication. This is an opportunity to lighten up the work day. Sometimes, for example, our staffers joke around by handing the person who "caught" them a type of candy they know the person doesn't like.

Try Candy and Stars . . . They Work!

It may sound kind of childish, but the strategy of changing behavior by awarding candy to staff who detect other staffers' lapses in procedures really works (see idea #13). We make it fun by adding an element of zaniness. In our pharmacy, it's not uncommon for the person who has earned a piece of candy to call out a request for a favorite flavor—and for the staffer who must deliver it to instead present a flavor that the person hates. We all get a kick out of it, and no one takes it too seriously.

In a similar vein, we recently had technicians give themselves stars on a poster board for greeting and offering help to patients who came into the pharmacy for reasons beyond getting prescriptions filled. At the end of the quarter, the technician with the most stars could select any of our pharmacists to pay for his or her lunch. What an incentive! Our company does telephone surveys to randomly selected patients to see if our customers get the attention they deserve. In that particular quarter, we scored "yes" on every question for a total of 100%. Because of these excellent results, we decided to buy pizza for the entire staff.

Idea #26 Obtain four pieces of information on all phone-in refills.

SEE RELATED IDEA #3, 20, 49, 76

Here is a simple idea to ensure consistency and quality. When prescription refills are phoned in to the pharmacy, be sure to ask patients:

1. Their prescription number. (Be sure they supply the correct number of digits!)

2. Their first and last name.

3. The approximate time they are coming in to pick up their prescription.

4. The phone number they are calling from, or where they can be reached if there are any problems.

Getting the patient's name is important because sometimes patients supply the wrong prescription number, they give you too many or too few digits, or the staff person taking the call writes the number down incorrectly. It doesn't do much good for the patient to tell you she is "Mrs. Barnabis" if you go to your computer and discover you have 15 people on file with the last name "Barnabis."

Knowing the approximate time a patient plans to arrive to pick up a prescription provides your staff with an extra tool for prioritizing workflow. Don't back yourselves into a corner by not obtaining information that is readily accessible.

Obtaining the prescription number is a no brainer. But getting this piece of information provides more opportunities than you'd think. When patients who call in for refills don't have their prescription number handy, look it up while you still have them on the phone. A vague statement from the patient like "please refill my dyazide" is simply too incomplete. Looking up the prescription number on the computer offers an excellent chance to detect problems and communicate refill status back to the patient. Perhaps the patient didn't clearly tell you which medication is needed, or maybe she got it at another pharmacy and it needs to be transferred.

Having the phone number, of course, allows you to reach the patient if there is a delay or a question about the prescription.

Don't Accept Unspecified Quantities

Here's a related thought—which also ties in with idea #3. Train your staff to never accept from patients an unspecified quantity change on a prescription refill. For example, what if a patient calls or comes into the pharmacy and says, "I need my medication, but I need double the amount." The last time that patient was in, he had also requested twice the amount, so the prescription was entered for a double fill. This time the patient is likely to receive four times the amount. Or what if the patient requests a half order? The last time her prescription was filled, the quantity dispensed was 30, so you give the patient 15 this time. But you don't realize that the previous time, the patient had also received one-half the amount of the original quantity ordered.

When patients start talking "one-half," "double," or some other vague amount, always ask them for the specific quantity. Otherwise, you've increased the chances that one of your staff will be redoing the refill to correct the error.

Taking a few extra seconds to get these four items while you have the caller on the phone can save you lots of time searching for them after you hang up. Write all four items on a slip of paper and place it on the very top of the colored basket referred to in idea #49. This way, the lead technician can easily scan the slips and continuously prioritize what needs to be filled. If you choose, you can include the four items on a "canned response" form similar to those described in idea #20. Idea #76 suggests three other pieces of information to obtain on prescriptions phoned in by the physician.

 Idea #27 Create a mission statement for your pharmacy.

A mission statement explains your reason for being in business. It is, quite simply, the reason your pharmacy exists. The following guide will assist you in creating your own unique mission statement.

Mission Statement

What business are you in? _____

_____

What markets (customers) do you serve? _____

_____

What products/services do you provide? _____

_____

What patient needs do you fulfill? _____

_____

What is your philosophy (standards and style) of doing business? _____

_____

An example of a mission statement might be:

"We are your experts in medication therapy. Our goal is to help you and all of our patients use and understand their medications with minimal side effects. We monitor your medications for safety and effectiveness. We want to make sure that you benefit from your medicine, and we will assist you with communicating to your doctor if any changes are necessary to improve your medicine's benefits to you. Preventing problems before they happen is best. We will consult with all patients about their medications, and help you in any way that we can."

If you work for a large chain, you may already have a corporate mission statement. Consider posting it. Also, don't be afraid to add to it if you feel it doesn't incorporate everything you are trying to accomplish.

Your Personal Mission Statement

From recent editorials in pharmacy journals, it's clear that some pharmacists are dissatisfied with their work environment. Creating your own professional mission statement is a way to initiate changes in your work environment that bring it more in line with your professional needs. Ask yourself these questions:

Why did I become a pharmacist? _____

_____

What do I believe my duties should be? Why? _____

_____

Jot the answers down and shape them into a mission statement now, while you're thinking about it.

If you wish, get input from others you work with before you finalize it. Then post your mission statement where you will see it every day. Consider sharing it with your supervisor.

Don't lose sight of your mission in life or why you thought pharmacy would be a great profession for you. You are a health care professional who deserves respect, and you have a right to practice in a way that helps improve others' lives. Tackle changes in your work environment that contribute to making your daily work compatible with your mission.

You can't do everything for everyone. Some current services may need to be eliminated. Major changes take time and persistence. Don't give up on them.

CHAPTER 4

"Don't be a slave to your in-box.

Just because something's there

doesn't mean you have to do it."

—Malcolm S. Forbes, Jr.

Tips for Managers and Supervisors

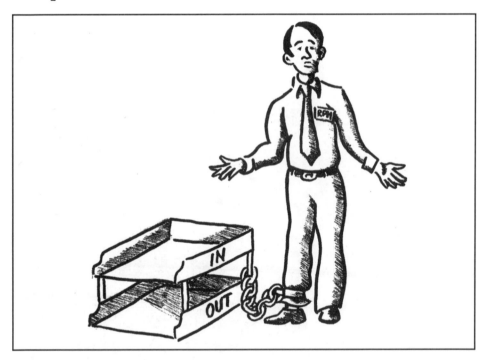

 Idea #28 Don't be a slave to your in-box.

How much information do you receive daily that has little or no value to you? Pharmacists seem to get inundated with material from every possible health-related mailing list. Here are some tips to help you sort through your mail and deal with it more efficiently.

A key tool for paper management is the TRAF method. I learned about it several years ago in a time management seminar. Here's how it works:

T - Throw it out! Just get rid of it immediately.

R - Refer it to someone else. Can it be delegated?

A - Act on it. Do something with it right now.

F - File it.

A tip I've found very helpful that relates to the "F" item is this: When deciding where to file something, ask yourself, "Where can I find this?" Most people tend to ask themselves, "Where should I put this?" Then it becomes a lost item.

Another great tip on filing is to ask yourself, "If I could not locate this piece of paper tomorrow, how much trouble would it cause for me?" If the answer is little or none, then throw it away. Using the TRAF system takes some practice. You may want to post it above or near your mailbox as a reminder.

Managing pharmacy journals and professional newsletters is a challenge, too. A good technique is to commit to reading one publication regularly that summarizes new information for you.

Another way to limit the amount of material you must absorb is to decide to specialize. Read only those articles related to one disease state. Most pharmacists are general practitioners; that is, they know a little bit about everything. Ask yourself which diseases you receive the most questions about and how you could be of the most help to your patients. Also consider whether one area of expertise might be more profitable than another.

Each time you look at a journal, imagine that you are a highly paid executive and your time is very valuable—so you must spend it wisely. Open the journal and look at the table of contents. Choose just one article to read in each journal. Circle the title and place the journal in an area designated "to read." If you don't get to it within two months, file the journal in one of those magazine holders available at many discount and office supply stores.

When possible, throw journals out after you read them. If you do save journals, limit your library to one year's worth or less. Chances are that after one year the information is either outdated or has appeared again in another journal. If you receive more than three monthly journals, consider canceling those you find least valuable.

When you want to save an article from a journal, don't keep the whole journal. Cut the article out, file it where you can find it (preferably a file on that subject), and throw the journal away.

At the end of your day, your in-box should be empty. Anything left to act on should be placed in a separate "to do" box. Items left in your in-box contribute to stress, the feeling that your job is never done or that you haven't accomplished anything. Keep your in-box cleared out.

 ### Idea #29 *Eliminate first party charges without affecting your business.*

Should we be taking a lesson from our colleagues in the prescription mail-order business? Prescriptions there must be paid for in advance by check or credit card. Not only are first party charges a source of bad debt, they also take up your time. With the number of third party programs and discount prescription cards increasing, profit margins are at an all-time low. It may be time to ask yourself whether to change your payment policy for prescriptions that you mail out.

Requesting that mail-out prescriptions be prepaid by credit card (or by check when customers do not have a credit card) will save you time and trouble. Fewer and fewer businesses allow customers to buy on credit anymore. Those that do are called Visa and MasterCard. And they charge 10% interest or more!

You could start by giving your patients six months' notice to anticipate the forthcoming change. Explain in your letter to patients that financial constraints have forced you to consider how you do prescription mail-outs. Note that you would like to be fair to everyone. Be sure you let them know how much you appreciate their business and emphasize that you would like to continue mailing their prescriptions. If the number of pharmacy patrons who buy from you on credit is small enough, explaining your new payment policy by telephone might help them better understand and accept it.

Difficult business decisions have to be made every day, and this is one of them. Obviously, if you work for someone else, you will have to get permission before proceeding with a plan to eliminate first party charges. Even if it doesn't work out exactly as planned and you decide to make a few exceptions for hardship cases, you will probably receive voluntary compliance from most people.

It might be encouraging to know that some pharmacies have actually decided to not accept third party insurance and have stayed in business—a much scarier prospect than eliminating customer charge accounts. They may have a niche business that includes prescription compounding or other sources of revenue, but even so, changing their payment policy so drastically must have been a difficult decision.

Tee Shirt Wisdom

A gentleman came into our pharmacy one day wearing a T-shirt that, on the front, advertised a certified public accounting firm. On the back it said, "In God we trust. Everyone else must pay cash!"

Idea #30 Solve problems by communicating.

The key to dealing with managers above you in the hierarchy is to be persistent, yet flexible. Your ideas and mine are not necessarily the solution to all of pharmacy's problems. The important thing is that you promote dialogue and open discussion. Avoid sounding like a whiner: If you bring up a problem, be prepared to offer solutions. Here are some ways to address issues in your work environment:

1. Communicate the problems you are having. Be clear and focused.

2. Talk to other pharmacists within your company to see if they are experiencing similar problems.

3. When you are proposing a solution, ask other pharmacists to voice their support for it at a district meeting or during their own visit with the supervisor.

4. Don't gang up or blind side the boss. Ask if there can be a place on the meeting agenda for your concerns.

5. Work on one major problem at a time.

6. When working to solve a problem, the following steps are useful:

- Ask for your supervisor's advice.
- Run your ideas by your supervisor.
- Get your supervisor's permission to take the action you are proposing.
- Have alternatives in mind in case an idea is rejected by your supervisor or, upon further reflection, seems unworkable.
- Push the limits of flexibility, be creative, and think outside of the box.

If you've followed these steps and feel like nothing has come of it, don't despair. Simply talking about an idea brings attention to it and causes it to be acknowledged. Months later the problem may be brought up again, and someone else may think they have a solution to it—the same solution you suggested. It doesn't matter who solves problems, as long as they are resolved. Sometimes I've been frustrated that solutions I've proposed seem to be ignored, but then time passes and all of a sudden, changes that are in line with my suggestions are enacted. Bureaucracies move slowly. But nothing will change at all if you never speak up about problems and ways to address them.

Question your own disbelief of what you think is possible. I would caution you not to force change, but rather push it along. Be positive.

 Idea #31 Use the "here's how we did it" approach.

A few years ago at a communication seminar I heard a story about a hospital surgery team that implemented a strategy to significantly reduce their patients' post-op recovery time. This strategy not only improved patients' satisfaction, but it saved money by decreasing the time that patients spent in the hospital after surgery. Elated by the results, two hospital administrators from different organizations sent their surgery teams to a presentation by the team that had made the discovery. One hospital administrator essentially ordered his team to put the same strategy into effect after they attended the presentation. The other administrator said, "Go and see what this is all about."

Well, the team that was directed to implement the change was resistant to doing so. The one that went simply to listen felt empowered to duplicate the new idea and produce the same results on their own. The moral of the story: If you allow people to discover the benefits of change on their own, they are more likely to embrace it.

When I learned several years ago that a pharmacy was using colored baskets to prioritize prescription orders, it seemed like a logical thing to do. I knew, though, that our staff would probably resist change. Instead of forcing it on them, I decided to try out the "here's how we did it" approach by simply describing that pharmacy's system to them while we were working. "When I was at the national pharmacy conference," I said, "I heard about a pharmacy that uses different colored baskets to organize their workflow. They use a white basket for patients who are waiting, a blue basket for patients coming later in the day, and a pink basket for mail outs." Then, about a half hour later I asked, "Do you guys think that idea would work here?"

Some mumbling took place. Not the resounding "yes!" I was hoping for, so I asked another question. "If we were to implement this idea in our pharmacy, what color baskets would you use?" Now we had a dialogue, and some differences of opinion. I asked if one of the technicians would like to go into the store and pick out some small basket trays to organize prescriptions. We started using the small baskets just to see what it was like, and agreed to try it for a couple weeks. The next day, the technicians explained the idea to the other pharmacy team members. A couple weeks later I asked, "Should we stop using the colored baskets now?" Jokingly they said, "Go away."

Idea #32 Meet basic human needs by taking adequate breaks.

At a recent pharmacy-related meeting, the topic of pharmacists' dedication to their patients came up. Several members of the group expressed the belief that pharmacists' commitment to serving patients causes them to sacrifice their own basic human needs, so that they do not take restroom breaks or stop to eat lunch when they need to. Contributing to this problem is the fact that leaving the pharmacy for five or ten minutes places pharmacists at a great disadvantage, because there is so much to catch up on when they return.

Doctors, nurses, and other health care professionals take lunch and go to the bathroom when necessary. In fact, just the other day I called over to the urgent care clinic with a question. I was told that the doctor and the nurse went to lunch, and would return in half an hour. What could be more urgent than urgent care, I wondered? Certainly not filling a prescription.

I decided to contact a urology office in town to find out what happens when people delay going to the restroom on a regular basis. "A series of fibrous bundles called 'trabeculae' can form on the inner lining of the bladder," the nurse replied. "This causes creases in the bladder, as the muscles are continuously overused. Eventually the bladder gets bigger and bigger. This leads to urinary frequency, and the inability to totally empty the bladder. It can be fixed," she said. "We just need to insert a super pubic catheter to rest the bladder muscle until it can shrink to its normal size."

"Sounds like fun," I replied. "Could you excuse me? I have to go to the bathroom right now."

In 1974, the U.S. Occupational Safety and Health Administration (OSHA) released a sanitation standard requiring employers to provide employees with toilet facilities. Although it appeared to be self-explanatory, apparently that wasn't the case. Therefore, in April 1998, the agency issued a memo to clarify its intent. OSHA's clarification was intended to ensure that employees do not experience adverse health effects (urinary tract infection, renal damage, constipation, abdominal pain, hemorrhoids, or diverticula) that can occur when they are unable to use (or are discouraged from using) the restroom.

Discussions between the American Pharmaceutical Association (APhA) and OSHA determined that, for the purposes of this regulation, pharmacists are employees. A federal interpretation stated, "Such access even includes providing relief workers for jobs in which even a brief absence could be disruptive." Since the release of this interpretation, OSHA has received questions from other professionals, including nurses and teachers. If you feel that your employer has broken this law and is unwilling to accommodate you, contact your regional OSHA office to report them.

If you work in an environment where taking a bathroom break puts a strain on your workflow, encourage your manager or district supervisor to discuss solutions to the problem at your next meeting. Also, find out if it is a problem with other pharmacists in your company. You may get better results if you are not the only one with this concern. But if you are, find out how those other pharmacists avoid the problem that is troubling you.

Idea #33 Have a weekly "meeting on paper."

SEE RELATED IDEA #21

What in the world is a meeting on paper, you ask? This is a strategy I read about in a time management book years ago. Quite simply, it's a memo.

Have you ever gone to a meeting where there were so many items on the agenda that you came away feeling overwhelmed? Or maybe you left the meeting just trying to remember half the things discussed. So many meetings have no impact on us because they try to cover too much in too short a time. We have regular meetings every other month from 8:00 am to 8:45 am. That's enough time for a couple of major topics and maybe one minor one, but it certainly isn't sufficient to explore every worthy issue that came up in the previous eight weeks.

One answer is to have a weekly meeting on paper (MOP). It should be limited to one page, everyone gets a copy, and no more than two to three topics are covered, such as information about new employees, drug recalls, and price changes. Explain to your staff what MOPs are before you start sending them. Essentially, they are a tool for making everyone's job a little easier.

Throughout the day when one of these memos is distributed, you can ask your staff what they thought about that morning's MOP. We encourage our staff to participate in impromptu discussions about each MOP so they have a better chance of remembering it.

By disseminating important information this way each week, your regular staff meetings will be shorter and more focused. Can you imagine how much more influential each meeting will be if your staff has to concentrate on only one or two topics? Then, if you follow up regular meetings with a written recap in each mailbox, you've got a well-informed staff.

Meeting on Paper

January 1, 2001

1. Insurance change. Beginning today, XYZ insurance company claims will be processed using a different group number. The old number was 1234. Please start using 5678, or claims may be rejected.

2. New drug. BeWell is a new medication on the market for depression. It comes in 10- and 20-mg tablets and is taken once a day.

3. Terminology adjustment. After discussions with many of you, we've decided it would be a good idea to refer to our customers as "patients." Our patients have come to know and respect us for helping them with their health and medications. Although they will always technically be our customers, we want to emphasize that we care for them as patients, and that we are health care providers.

 Idea #34 Schedule some technicians in six-hour shifts to save time on breaks and lunch.

For years, we scheduled technicians in eight-hour shifts. Their routine: work two hours, take a 15-minute break (paid), work two more hours, take a 30-minute lunch (unpaid), work two more hours, and then take another 15-minute break (paid). You know it all too well.

Then we got an idea. If we scheduled some of our technicians for six hours instead of eight, we would save 45 minutes per person in breaks and lunches, because by law we would only have to give them one 15-minute break. In a large-volume store we could save one and a half to three hours per day, or 30 to 60 hours a month in payroll. (If your state law is different regarding how long an employee can work before taking a lunch, you will have to follow those laws.)

This savings may not sound like much, but think about it. Such a schedule keeps the workflow going because fewer breaks must be accommodated. It's almost like having a technician come in at mid-day and provide 45 minutes of "catch-up" work to help reduce the staff's workload and stress.

Because the pharmacy business requires us to work nights and week-ends, it demands that we have full accessibility to our staff whenever the pharmacy is open. With eight-hour shifts, having a working crew of four technicians only amounts to three and a half technicians, because somebody is always on break or at lunch. That's a 12.5% reduction in your daily work force, regardless of how many techni-cians you have scheduled.

You may think that your employees won't like working six-hour shifts, or will not be happy about being given less than 40 hours per week. But you may be surprised by how many jump at the chance to be home when their children get out of school, or want to reduce their hours for some other reason. Test the amount of interest in six-hour shifts by asking for volunteers. Many of our employees found that they like having an extra two and a half hours of free time in their day for the price of two—since they aren't forced by law to take an unpaid lunch break in the middle of a six-hour shift.

You can give technicians just one or two six-hour shifts per week to start. Your technicians will still work 36 to 38 hours per week. You'll find that those on a lighter schedule are much more willing to stay a little extra if needed, and you don't have to pay them overtime.

We tried this approach for 60 days to give it a fair chance, and now we have technicians who volunteer eagerly for six-hour shifts. If you try it once and it doesn't work out, it may be wise to try it again in three months. People's personal lives and needs change. You may find that an idea that originally met with resistance is no longer unpopular.

We still schedule some eight-hour shifts when there is low technician supply, high prescription demand, or both, but for every six-hour shift we have added an extra 45 minutes to our work day. Keep an open mind. Consider allowing a one-hour scheduling gap, if your business volume will accommodate it. For example, change your two shifts so that instead of 9 am–5 pm and 5 pm–9 pm, technicians are scheduled 9 am–3 pm and 4 pm–9 pm. Your pharmacy's hours of operation may differ from this example, but if you experiment and play around with the schedule a bit, you should find a formula that works for you.

Idea #35 Emphasize that you are a health care professional.

Rather than viewing one's self as being in a customer service profession with a health care component, improve your own job satisfaction and morale by communicating regularly to your superiors that you are a health care professional first, with a customer service component.

As health care professionals, we have a responsibility to our patients, but because we dispense a product, some upper-level managers perceive our role as "customer service" rather than "patient care." Do not fall into this trap. Regularly get across the message to managers that you—and pharmacists in general—are health care professionals first, but happen to handle customer service, too.

Like nurses, we extend the care provided by physicians and play an integral role in patients' health. But our functions differ from those of nurses because we monitor patients' drug therapy and carry out interventions that result in improved medication safety and better outcomes. To help other managers understand this concept, provide them copies of journal articles regarding pharmacists' professional services. Pharmacists who do not stand up for their rights as health care professionals are cheating the patient, the profession, and themselves out of a career that should be rewarding and enjoyable.

Always communicate with superiors in your organization in a professional, respectful way. If you decide to change jobs or are ever in need of a reference, you might need the help of a former boss or employer, so never burn bridges. This advice applies to all pharmacists—whether you are a manager or not.

Not burning bridges, however, does not mean failing to stand up for your rights as a person, manager, or health care professional. You have human needs, such as restroom breaks and lunches, as well as professional needs, such as putting your skills to use. You have a right to help people with their medication-related problems, as opposed to spending your time counting by fives as quickly as you can.

> "You may have to fight a battle
> more than once to win."
>
> —Margaret Thatcher

CHAPTER 5

"Few things

are impossible to

diligence and skill."

—Samuel Johnson

Taking Control of Your Work Day

Idea #36 Redirect long-winded patients.

Helping long-winded patients can be a virtue when time allows, but during a prescription storm it can send stress levels to new heights. Long-winded patients appear on the telephone, in the over-the-counter (OTC) section, and at prescription windows. They mean well, but sometimes have difficulty focusing on the intended question. You can draw upon a couple of great techniques when you're tied up with a long-winded patient and there seems no way out.

Canned responses, such as those discussed in idea #20, can help you focus or redirect the patient. When you need to wrap things up with long-winded patients on the telephone, try interjecting the questions below. Post them—or others you create that suit you better—by the phone until you are comfortable using them.

1. "Now, what was your question?"
2. "Mrs. Baker, did you have a specific question in mind?"
3. "Mr. Simpson, do you have any more questions today?"
4. "Can you hold, please?"
5. "Can I call you back?"

I call the first two "director" questions. They are intended to direct the conversation from mere discussion to an endpoint—the question. The third question is useful when patients have already explained to you what they need to know, but they continue to elaborate. Questions four and five can be introduced this way:

"Mrs. Johnson, I have a couple of patients waiting for me at the consultation window. Can you hold, please? Or can I call you back?" Often patients will reply that they have no further questions, and will simply thank you for your time. You can add some frosting to the service cake by thanking patients for calling and reminding them that if they have further questions, they are welcome to call anytime.

When you encounter long-winded patients in the OTC section, you're most likely helping them select a product. Once you've made a recommendation, patients may study the product label or compare ingredients and prices of several products in that category. They don't really need your help at the moment, but you might feel uncomfortable walking away. These two "exit statements" allow you to leave without sounding rude.

1. "I'll be right over here. If you have any more questions, just let me know."

2. "If you'll excuse me, I have a prescription to finish. Please let me know if I can be of more assistance."

Probably the most difficult situation to walk away from politely is when a patient is standing directly in front of you at the prescription counter. The two statements above generally work well. If patients tie up your time regularly at the prescription counter, post these—and other responses you feel comfortable using—somewhere convenient for reference.

Idea #37 Use an OTC consultation form.

We started using the form on the next page when we noticed we were too busy to perform our professional prescription-related duties effectively and still provide adequate consultation on over-the-counter (OTC) products. We wanted to give the same professional attention to patients in the OTC section as those who have prescriptions—after all, both come to us because of a health care need. And we recognized that the large number of Rx to OTC switches in the last several years yields a great opportunity for us to provide basic pharmaceutical care.

OTC Consultation Form

Patient is: Myself   Spouse   Child   Parent   Other:_____

            Male   Female   Symptoms started (date) _____

            Age: _____

Prescription medications this person is taking: Prednisone? Coumadin/Warfarin?

_____   _____   _____   _____

_____   _____   _____   _____

Over-the-counter medications this person is taking:

_____   _____   _____   _____

Have you tried anything for today's problem already?

_____   _____   _____   _____

List any medical history or doctor's diagnosis for this person:

    Heart (Describe) _____

High blood pressure	Asthma	Emphysema	High thyroid
Diabetes:	Insulin?	Oral medication?	Prostate problem
Difficulty urinating	Trouble sleeping	Surgery	

    Others not listed here: _____

Symptoms

Aches or pains	Stuffy nose	Sneezing	Headache
Sinus congestion	Runny nose/ Nasal drainage	Sore throat	Cough
Itchy or watery eyes	Sinus pressure	Swelling	Ears are plugged
Chest congestion	Pain or ringing in ears	High fever	Fever

Thank you!

This form helps tremendously when you don't have time to gather an adequate patient history. It's a relatively quick and concise method for maximizing your efficiency. After the patient fills out the form, you review it with them to be sure you understand all the information and are ready to make a recommendation. Feel free to copy the supplied form and use it as is, or modify it to meet your own needs.

Idea #38 Put drugs away using basket organizers.

We used to run to our five shelving bays several times a day to put drug orders away. We would grab three, four, or sometimes five bottles at a time to speed up the process. Then one day we discovered that another pharmacy used a special basket for each bay to put their drugs away, and we decided to adopt the same procedure. The baskets we use measure about 10 inches wide by 12 inches long and 8 inches deep. They're available at many department and discount stores.

Now a technician can take the basket into the bay area and not have to make 70 or 80 trips back and forth. Five trips and the entire order is on the shelves.

We could have had a meeting to discuss the running-back-and-forth problem, propose the basket solution, allow people to express their concerns, and listen to reasons why the baskets wouldn't work, but why go there? Using baskets is a thing we just did, on the spot, that very day.

Of course, when you change something that you've always done one way, invariably there will be setbacks, such as the temptation to revert to old procedures that are deeply ingrained. The key is to commit to the change and keep tweaking your new approach until it works for you.

Idea #39 Do not provide services for free.

Think about all that's involved in filling a prescription. Here's the short version: You provide patients with all the services mandated under the Omnibus Budget Reconciliation Act of 1990 (OBRA '90), and what you get in return is average wholesale price (AWP) - 15% + $1.75.

Now for the long version of what you do when you fill a prescription:

- Interpret the prescription order
- Do a patient intake history
- Input information into the computer
- Count pills
- Label the bottle
- Attach warning labels
- Ensure accuracy of the order
- Scan patient profile for drug interactions
- Check patient profile for allergies
- Consult with physician if necessary to resolve problems with the prescription
- Perform a final check of the prescription
- Talk with patient to clarify the drug's indication
- Explain to patient how to take the medication
- Explain to patient which side effects to watch for
- Explain to patient how to know if the medication is working
- Answer patient's questions
- Provide printed information leaflets, if applicable
- Solve insurance problems
- Smile
- Say thank you

Years ago, pharmacy staff had the time and pharmacies had the money to do little extras for patients free of charge. But today, insurance companies have squeezed profit margins to an all-time low.

Ask yourself this question: Are we providing free services that could be charged for? These services may not, by definition, be true "pharmaceutical care," but many kinds of assistance we offer patients warrant a small fee to cover our time—which is valuable and limited. Some possibilities to consider:

Tablet splitting ....$1.50 for 30

Prefilling insulin syringes...$1.00 each

Diabetes monitor training...$30.00

Blood glucose monitor services:

Basic cleaning $5.00

Troubleshooting... $5.00–$15.00

Blood sugar screening $12.00

Computerized diabetes data management printouts $16.00

Above with consultation..$34.00

Therapeutic substitution cost-savings
analysis for cash-paying patients.............20% of first year's savings

Peak flow meter training..$16.00

In thinking about how to communicate these fees, consider what other professionals might do. For example, for basic diabetes monitor cleaning or troubleshooting, you could create a form on which you provide an estimate of fees. Tell the patient, "I'll have to fill out a service order for this. Please initial by the estimate."

A Lesson in Sales

My Uncle Myron was in the television repair business. He used to say that a good salesman always tells customers they will have to leave the T.V. set at the shop for a couple days, even if the problem is something that can be fixed immediately. "There's no perceived value if the customer isn't without the product for a day or two," he would explain.

Leaving a diabetes monitor at the pharmacy for two days would be excessive, but maybe pharmacists could tell patients that they need to leave the monitor for a couple hours until there's a chance to service it. This is a way to combat the "we do it all for you right now" mentality that has gotten pharmacists overwhelmed by an unmanageable workload.

Idea #40 Require 24 hours' notice for all compounded prescriptions.

Next to third party insurance problems, compounding prescriptions tops the list of things that interrupt the pharmacist's work day. If the bulk of your business involves dispensing products from the manufacturer's bottle—and if you are the only pharmacist on duty—you're not prepared for an interruption of 15 minutes or more to compound a prescription on the spot.

Instead, establish a policy stating that compounded prescriptions require 24 hours for completion.

Depending on how busy you are at the time, you may want to try to fill a patient's first compounded prescription the same day they bring it in. They may live far from your pharmacy and may need the initial prescription right away. A quick turnaround the first time prevents patients from taking the prescription elsewhere. At the same time, you can notify them that you generally ask for 24 hours' notice for compounding.

To help meet the needs of patients who have not given you 24 hours' notice, offer to call them when their compounded medication is ready to pick up. Another option is to have patients prepay the prescription so you can mail it out when it is ready. Although mailing will take a few days, it's still a reasonable time frame when you consider that some managed care mail order companies take 10 to 14 business days (that's two to three weeks!) to mail out new prescriptions.

CHAPTER 6

"When one door of happiness closes, another opens;

but we often look so long at the closed door,

that we do not see the one which has opened for us."

—Helen Keller

The New Art of Delegating

Idea #41 Condition patients to call their doctors for refills.

One of the most important things we have done to reduce stress and increase professionalism in the pharmacy is to stop calling doctors for refills. No, we haven't stopped completely—we still call on behalf of some patients who are in special circumstances—but most of our patients have been conditioned to call on their own.

I have seen both chain and independent pharmacies successfully put the responsibility on patients to call doctors for refills. This strategy, however, creates controversy among pharmacists. Some believe that patients will stop taking their medications if pharmacists don't call doctors for refills. To such pharmacists, I ask the question, what will the patient do when his or her physician insists that the patient come in for an appointment before yet another refill can be authorized? Physicians can't keep refilling prescriptions indefinitely over the phone—they must see patients in person periodically. By continuing to call doctors for refills on behalf of patients, pharmacists are essentially hindering patients from taking responsibility for their own health.

A physician at a major clinic in our area insists that his patients get all their prescriptions refilled when they visit him. While the patient is still at the clinic he either writes a new prescription for them or phones in a refill to the pharmacy. The clinic also has signs posted throughout the waiting and examination rooms telling patients to bring all their prescription bottles to every doctor appointment. This physician is tired of being interrupted throughout the day to authorize refills. Pharmacists could learn a lot about time management from him.

The same doctor once left the following message (word for word) on our voice mail. "I'm calling in a prescription for a patient of Dr. Jones for a Flovent inhaler. I hope she got it there before, because she didn't tell me the strength of it, and I'm not going to waste my time pulling her chart up. So please give her whatever strength inhaler she had before, one time, and she can get the rest of the refills from Dr. Jones. Not on the weekend. Thank you very much. Good-bye!" I must admit, I found his comments a little harsh. But I believe that other physicians and pharmacists share some of the frustration he expressed.

Some physicians' offices have placed responsibility on the pharmacies they associate with to handle the time-consuming refill procedure. See Idea #77 for ways to change this expectation. A pharmacy in our town uses the fax machine to streamline the refill process and incorporate it into their workflow, which works well for them. They simply print the prescription refill screen, circle the important data, write a short message requesting authorization for refills, and fax it to the physician's office. This still takes valuable pharmacy time, but is a compromise the pharmacy is willing to make.

Delegating to patients the responsibility for initiating prescription refill authorizations has distinct advantages for the patient, physician, and pharmacy. It's a "win-win-win" strategy, because it benefits everyone involved—especially patients. After all, whom do we work for? Isn't it more advantageous to patients if we focus our energy on professional functions that help improve their health? When we spend too much time on one patient—especially handling a routine technical function like calling a doctor about a prescription refill—it's at the expense of everyone else.

We decided to change the process in our pharmacy partly because we came to believe that when the pharmacy initiates the refill, it contributes to our nation's problem of patient noncompliance. In other words, it encourages patients to be complacent. If patients have to look at their prescription bottle, they are forced to read the name, strength, and directions. This increases their understanding of their medication and promotes a more active role in their therapy. We want to empower patients to take ownership of and responsibility for their health care. Some other reasons for making the change:

- When pharmacies call the doctor's office for refills, insurance delays can occur if the doctor's staff does not pull the chart and provide specifics. The label directions may turn out to be incorrect if we base them on outdated pharmacy information. Eventually, the insurance company may reject the claim as "refill too soon"—which could be averted if patients were to contact their physicians *directly* for refills.

- Patients often get through to the doctor just as quickly as pharmacists do, so there is no overall time advantage in having pharmacists call. Plus, when pharmacists make the call, patients lose sight of the fact that it takes time. Thus they get angry at the pharmacist if their prescription isn't ready when they think it should be. Since we changed our approach, we've seen a reduction in patients who become hostile because they expect an expired refill to be ready for them before their doctor even calls us back.

- It reduces the amount of paper floating around as well as miscellaneous follow-up notes.

- It prevents the pharmacist from becoming the "middle man," delivering messages back and forth.

- It cuts down the pharmacist's telephone load without increasing the number of calls the patient or doctor must make. If the patient contacts the physician's office for refill authorization, and the physician calls the pharmacy, that's one call for the patient, two for the physician, and one for the pharmacy. If, on the other hand, the patient calls the pharmacy, the pharmacy must still call the doctor, who will call the pharmacy back. That's one call for the patient, and two for the doctor, but it's three for the pharmacy.

- It lowers stress for everyone in the pharmacy and frees up valuable time for professional functions like pharmaceutical care and patient counseling. In the long run, it may reduce workload, improve department morale, and help attract quality pharmacists.

Here's what we did to retrain patients to call for their own prescription refills—a process I call "the new art of delegation":

1. We established a six-month window—a "grace period," if you will—during which we would still call for refills if the patient requested. We figured that half a year was plenty of time to allow patients to get used to the change. During the grace period, we made exceptions when patients insisted that we call the physician, and we'd make a note in the patient's files if special circumstances warranted that the pharmacy make the call. For example, we still call for a couple of our patients who have Alzheimer's disease, and also for one with a speech problem.

2. We scripted responses that we could easily refer to when discussing our new procedure with patients. Some staffers found it very difficult to convey this information, and we wanted it to be communicated positively. We posted our responses by each phone and by the patient intake window in the pharmacy.

3. If a patient called on the phone for a refill and we discovered the refills were expired when we went to process the prescription, we would call the patient right back. Typical of what we might say is: "Mrs. Jones, did you realize that your prescription has no more refills on it? . . . Do you have a new prescription from your doctor? . . . No? . . . What you will need to do, then, is call your doctor and have her update your prescription. If you are completely out of your medicine, we could give you a couple of tablets to hold you over until your doctor calls in the refill."

4. If patients came into the pharmacy without realizing their prescription had expired we'd offer to give them a couple days' worth of medication to last until they could reach their physician. A simple note in the computer allows us to subtract from the patient's next refill quantity the one or two days' supply we've provided to

hold the patient over. We also allow patients to use our phone if they would like to call their doctor from the pharmacy. One of the higher-volume pharmacies in our company used to have a phone designated for patient use at the cash register.

5. When patients objected to our request that they call their physician, we would kindly explain that we do not get through to their doctor any faster than they do; like them, we get the receptionist. We would also explain that they don't necessarily have to make an appointment with their doctor to receive a refill—the nurse might simply ask how they are doing. But if the patient insisted, we would make the call.

Even Partial Success Is Good

If you can't seem to take this strategy beyond point number 3, consider yourself successful even if *some* patients agree to take responsibility for their own refills.

You may be thinking about this idea, "We can't do that," "It won't work here," or "Not in my area!" I used to feel the same way. It's a strategy that represents "out-of-the-box" thinking, which tends to spark controversy and objection. What I've learned is that if a new idea doesn't cause you to step back and say, "yeah, right," then you're not thinking outside of the box.

There's no question—this strategy has been critical in freeing up our pharmacists' time to practice more professionally. Interestingly, the August 21, 2000 issue of *Drug Topics* reports that a new law in North Carolina prevents insurance companies from requiring pharmacists to call them for patients when a problem arises, because it takes too much of the pharmacist's time.

I can honestly say that not one patient has left our pharmacy because of our change in approach. One of our patients insisted we keep calling his doctor because, he said, "It's a long-distance call" for him. We agreed, and when he next came into the pharmacy I made a point to get to know him better. About a year later, one of our other pharmacists commented, "I don't think Mr. Anderson has actually requested that we call in his refills since you first talked to him about it."

"No," I said, "I think he just wanted to know that we would do it for him if he asked us to."

When we retrieve refill requests from our touch tone telephone refill system and find that the prescription the patient is calling about has expired, we call him or her back as soon as possible. Many times, when we reach these patients, they are very apologetic. Before we even do anything more than identify ourselves, they tell us they've called their doctor or will be calling shortly. (Our touch tone system notifies callers, after they type in their prescription number, whether their refills have expired.) Now they are conditioned to take care of this task themselves.

Conditioning patients to call their doctor for refills has probably freed up more of our time than anything else we've done—and everyone has benefited.

Idea #42 Hand the patient the phone right in the pharmacy.

Handing patients our phone right in the pharmacy when they need refill authorization from a doctor or are having insurance problems has proven to be a time-saving tool we never would have considered in the past. A key benefit is that it allows us to help such

SEE RELATED IDEA #43, 57

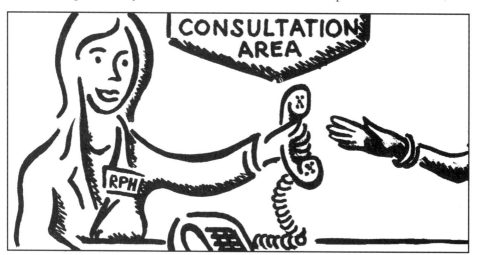

patients without abandoning everyone else. The pharmacist is always no more than five steps away if the patient holding the phone needs assistance.

By offering to dial patients' insurance companies and then handing them the phone, we help patients help themselves. We aren't deserting them. We let them know that we will be assisting other patients and we emphasize that once they have someone from the insurance company on the line, we're happy to jump in if they need us to explain something. Meanwhile, the patient is listening to "Endless Love" on hold, while we're tending to other patients. Every five minutes or so we check back with the patient to "see how things are going."

Some benefits of involving the patient in the problem-solving process this way:

- It's a convenience for the patient to be able to use the pharmacy's phone.

- The patient has a better understanding of the refill process when the receptionist says, "I'll need to pull your chart and have the doctor call it in later."

- Patients gain understanding of the third party voice mail maze. They realize that reasons entirely out of the pharmacy's control can delay their prescription.

- It keeps the pharmacist from being the middleman and the one who has to relay bad news. The patient's frustration about the problem is redirected from the pharmacist to the insurance company, or whoever the patient is calling.

- It allows patients to take ownership of their health care needs.

- Patients often need to contact their employee benefits department to resolve insurance-related problems; it's not something the pharmacist can take care of for them.

Think about it. You're still helping the patient solve the problem, but you're avoiding being stuck on hold yourself while the work piles up. Even if you were to have a technician or clerk make the call, it reduces your staff by one person, and everyone else must pick up the slack.

Why should pharmacists operate in a manner so out of sync with the rest of the world? Doctors and nurses are not responsible for procuring payment for their services, and neither is the receptionist. Clinics and doctors' offices have a billing department to deal with insurance companies, and that department forwards the bill to the patient for reconciliation if the insurance doesn't pay. When you go to a restaurant, who's responsible if your credit card doesn't go through? You are.

Since initiating this approach we've found that patients perceive us as having done everything we can for them, simply because we offer "assistance"—that is, we hand them the phone. The really great thing is that, in the end, the patient still likes us, which was not the case when we tried to solve insurance problems for them.

Idea #43 Delegate third party problems to the patient with ease.

When we receive an insurance rejection, we politely let the patient know we are having trouble processing their claim and we need their help. We never tell them they were "rejected" by their insurance company. To avoid that word, which has a negative connotation, we say, "Your prescription claim is not going through today for some reason. Do you have any idea why?" Then we add, "You will need to contact your insurance company or your employee benefits department. Would you like me to dial for you?" We hand them the receiver and the base of telephone in case they must push buttons in response to a voice mail system.

Ask the patient to document the first and last name of the person they speak with at the insurance company, as well as the person's direct phone number, so you can track him or her down later if you need to verify anything.

Sometimes, if we anticipate a quick resolution, we make the call for the patient instead of handing him or her the phone. But if we become trapped in a voice mail maze, we kindly ask the patient to hold the

---

line for us while we help other patients, as explained in idea #42. No one has ever refused to do it. (For tips on how to argue on behalf of the patient if you must talk with the insurance company, see idea #57.)

Always give the patient choices. In our pharmacy the other day, I overheard a technician explaining to a patient that her insurance card wasn't going through. The technician asked if the patient "would like to call her insurance company and come back later, or pay cash and return in a couple days to resubmit the claim." Both solutions the technician proposed were solution-based and prevented the pharmacy staff's time from being tied up, which would have delayed prescriptions for many other patients.

Idea #44 Have technicians order all drugs.

Ordering drugs is not a function that has to be done by a pharmacist. It can be delegated to a technician.

A few years ago, we were closed-minded and didn't think a technician could do an effective job ordering medications. It was too easy to say, "See, they made a mistake." But like anything else, it takes training and practice.

Once we made the decision to go forward, it didn't take long before technicians were doing all the ordering. They now order from our daily wholesaler or directly from manufacturers, and they take care of all special-order over-the-counter items. They also handle wholesaler returns, drug recalls, and outdated items.

Idea #45 Change the way you handle vacation supplies.

Since the advent of pharmacy benefits managers (PBMs), patients' requests for a vacation supply of prescription medications invariably cause problems. Pharmacists often find themselves in a difficult position, because patients can't get the amount they need to carry them through their vacation. What do you do?

We used to spend a lot of time trying to get through to the insurance company. Sometimes the responses we received from companies suggested that they didn't much care whether our patients had enough medication to last through vacation or not. Then it would fall to the pharmacist or technician to tell the patient, "Sorry, we can't fill it." The wasted time and the anger expressed by the patient affected morale and our ability to help others. Finally we decided to change our procedure.

Now, if an insurance company doesn't allow an override that lets the prescription be refilled early, before the patient leaves on vacation, the patient has two choices.

1. They can pay cash and submit their claim to the insurance company manually.

2. They can use our phone to contact the insurance company. We explain to the patient that when the pharmacy staff calls, we often get rejected. When patients call they might have better luck, since they are the ones paying for the insurance policy.

With this approach, no time is lost by anyone on the pharmacy staff and if the patient is upset, it is always at the insurance company. It might even prompt patients to complain to their employer about the PBM, which could result in a change to their policy regarding vacation supplies.

Idea #46 Stop trying to figure out the best deal on third party discount cards.

Third party discount cards have become so prevalent that patients often bring in two or three wanting to know which one is the best deal. We used to run each card through, then cancel each transaction, and rerun the card that saved the patient the most money. Every time we did this, we incurred a processing fee from the third party switching service. It took up our time, and all we got for our trouble was the average wholesale price minus a discount.

Now we tell patients we don't really know which is the better deal. "The price should be about the same at any pharmacy," we explain, "but the only way to find out what it would cost at our end is to create a false claim, then cancel it and create another false claim." We note that the plan sponsor should be able to state what the prescription will cost.

We also warn patients, "Be cautious if the sponsor is charging a fee." Many discount prescription cards charge a monthly membership fee, so they end up costing patients more than if patients simply paid the usual and customary price for prescription medications. Plus these cards do nothing to support professional pharmacy services, because they cut so deeply into profitability.

Imagine if a company came along that said, "Pay me $7.95 a month, and I'll give you a card that will save you 50 cents a gallon on gasoline." That's how these prescription discount cards work. But then what would happen is this: Your neighborhood gas station starts giving terrible service and can't afford enough employees because these cards are cutting into its profits. I've been told that, because of the problems prescription discount cards cause, at least one national chain pharmacy refuses to accept them.

It's not a bad idea to let patients with third party discount cards know that the companies issuing them have access to their medical information and could potentially sell it to pharmaceutical companies or marketing firms to make money. People need to be concerned about the privacy of their records. Pharmacists realize that true insurance companies have access to this information, too, but they have a measure of confidence that the patient's privacy will be protected. When cards are not backed by true insurance companies, there is no regulatory body overseeing how they operate or use the information they receive. Information about an AIDS patient could be revealed to an employer, or information about a person's cardiac risk could end up with an insurance company.

Sometimes patients with two active discount cards ask us to use the best card for each individual medication they are picking up. The difference in savings is usually only a few cents. We explain to patients that they need to choose one card or the other, because otherwise we are creating false claims. We tell them we will be happy (as far as they know) to accept either one. Gone are the days where we spend time analyzing the best deal on prescription discount cards.

If a patient asks you, "What discount will this card give me, and is it better than my old card?" the best response is, "That's a good question. I really don't know, ma'am. You would need to call the insurance company to find out. The number for your insurance company is on the back of your card." We always say this with genuine concern and kindness. (See idea #18 for tips on positive communication.)

Idea #47 Use technicians' help with prescription transfers.

Many states don't allow technicians to actually transfer a prescription to another pharmacy. This doesn't mean, however, that technicians can't carry out the technical functions that are involved.

When I call another pharmacy to arrange for a prescription transfer, I'm always pleased when technicians answer the phone, but often disappointed with their responses. Typically their answer to my request for a transfer is, "Just a minute and I'll get the pharmacist."

In a work environment that uses technicians effectively, I would expect to hear this: "If you will provide me with the patient's name and prescription number, I will pull the prescription hard copy for the pharmacist and bring it up on the computer screen. I'll also take your name, phone number, and the name of the pharmacy you're calling from to give to the pharmacist to document."

In states that allow technicians to document the transfer electronically after the pharmacist has given the transfer, the transfer information could be handed back to the technician to complete. If the technician is busy, the transfer information could be placed in a basket for him or her to complete when time permits.

Make a list of steps you expect technicians to follow when requests come in for prescription transfers (see box, next page). Post the list by the phone with the other "canned responses" you've developed, to be sure you get all the information you need. Delegating the management of prescription transfers to technicians is easy if you give them a protocol to follow.

Directions to Technicians for Handling Prescription Transfers

- When requests come in for prescription transfers, technicians should ask the caller for the following:

  — Prescription number

  — Patient name

  — Pharmacy name

  — Pharmacy phone number

  — Pharmacist's name

- Pull the prescription hard copy for the pharmacist (if necessary) and bring the prescription up on the computer screen.

CHAPTER 7

"Don't put that

monkey on my back."

—Traditional Saying

Workflow

 Idea #48 Clear all clutter.

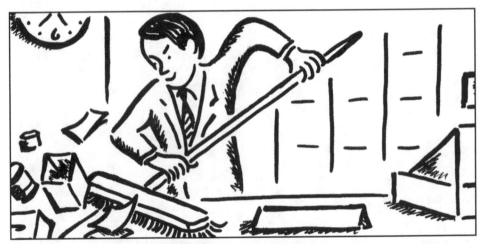

Other peoples' perceptions of you and the services you perform are linked to the appearance of your work environment. That's an important reason to get rid of clutter. You don't want your patients to judge you as messy and disorganized. Another reason is that an untidy workspace can make you less effective in carrying out your tasks.

First, take down all sticky notes from walls, counters, and computer terminals, and consolidate all the information they contain onto one easy-to-read sheet of paper. If you don't use the information daily, place it in a binder nearby.

Take a good look around. When was the last time you took everything off your workspace? Get rid of rubber stamps you no longer use, miscellaneous paper clips and rubber bands, and paper pads. The rule of thumb is, if you don't use it every day, it doesn't belong there.

Consider putting your prescription balance in a cupboard if you don't use it daily. How does the sink area look? Does the carpet get vacuumed regularly? These are all things that make for a harried work environment and contribute to stress. They are constant reminders that you always need to do more and that your job is never done.

Remove old posters from the walls and scrape off remnants of tape. How many cardboard advertisements do you have on top of your counters? These items start to look like junk after a while. We have eliminated all drug manufacturers' propaganda from our counter tops, something I advise you to try. And you probably don't need those little stands that say "We accept this or that insurance plan," do you?

A former salesman with marketing experience told me that to get a message across to the consumer, you have to limit yourself to one or two points. The one message we highlight is our "bunny service," described in idea #7. We want our patients to recognize that their health and welfare are number one on our list.

Go out into your pharmacy and take a birds-eye view of what the patient sees. Does the pharmacy appear clean and neat? Does it come across as the environment of health professionals? Are you sending a clear message about who you are and what you do? If not, decide what to change to convey the message you want.

Idea #49 Prioritize prescriptions using colored baskets.

SEE RELATED IDEA #5, 38

We use colored prescription baskets to organize prescription orders according to how soon they must be filled. Such baskets can be purchased inexpensively at many discount and office supply stores. I recommend three different colors. We use white, blue, and maroon. Our baskets are about 9 inches long, 5 inches wide, and 3 inches deep.

The baskets are situated near the prescription intake window so it's convenient to put processed prescriptions in them. As we receive each prescription order or refill request slip, it goes into the basket immediately so the lead technician can prioritize it. If there are multiple prescriptions for different people in the same family, they all go together as one order.

Here's our system:

- The white basket is the "priority" basket. It holds prescription orders and completed prescriptions for patients who are in the pharmacy waiting for them or who will arrive in the next two hours to pick up their medications. When time allows, we always try to complete prescriptions first for patients who are waiting on site, and we do the call-in prescriptions next.

- The blue basket is mostly for call-ahead prescriptions. When patients tell us that their approximate pickup time will be more than two hours later, their order and their completed prescription go into a blue basket.

- The maroon basket is for prescriptions that will be picked up the next day or will be mailed out. They are low priority and get done last. We may also use this basket for prescriptions that are being placed on hold to be filled on another date, if the patient doesn't need it now.

Once a basket makes it to the cash register area, the medication is placed in a bag and filed alphabetically for pickup, as in most pharmacies.

You may want to add a fourth basket in another color to designate prescriptions that must be delivered, and even a fifth to indicate "highest priority," as in our "bunny service" concept.

This idea, which I picked up at a professional pharmacy meeting, has served us well for over five years. Some pharmacists and technicians had a hard time with it at first, but once they used the system for a few weeks, they couldn't imagine going back to the old way.

 ### Idea #50 *Write the intake time on all new prescriptions.*

SEE RELATED IDEA #26

If you have the intake time—the time a prescription order was dropped off—written on the face of the prescription order, it gives you a mechanism for prioritizing prescriptions. We have a tiny digital clock sitting on the computer terminal stand, in plain view of the person taking the prescription order, so he or she can easily note the time.

If a prescription is delayed for some reason, such as the need to deal with an insurance problem or clarify information with the physician, having the intake time on it allows you to place it back into the workflow in the order it was received. Noting the intake time also allows you to gauge how long the prescription wait has been. If you are telling patients the wait is 10 to 15 minutes, and it's turning out to be 20 minutes, you can adjust what you say to patients dropping off prescriptions. Giving patients a realistic wait time is important.

Harold Goldstein, MD
DEA# AS1234567

3:52 p.m.

Internal Medicine
300 Medical Way
Hometown, NY 12200
513-244-5556

NAME *Susan Smith*

ADDRESS _____ DATE *5/30/00*

℞

Fioricet, plain

disp # 20

ī - īī Q 4-6 L paw

headache.

☑ Label

Refill ___/___ times   PRN   NR

H. Gold _____ M.D.

To insure brand name dispensing, prescriber must write 'Brand Necessary' or 'Brand Medically Necessary' on the prescription.

Have Technicians Verify Information

To avoid long delays and angry patients, it's helpful to verify information on new prescriptions patients drop off, before they walk away. We always ask for:

- Their name and spelling.

- Date of birth.

- Allergies to medications. (This information may have changed since their last visit, so we always ask.)

- The doctor's name and the spelling, if necessary.

We used to clarify only one or two of these items and ignore the rest. But it seemed like we were always calling patients back into the pharmacy. Now we take a few extra seconds up front, and it has proved to be a worthwhile investment of our time.

Idea #51 Have technicians fill all prescriptions.

SEE RELATED IDEA #24, 52

Many pharmacies have already revamped their systems so that technicians do all the filling. But some are held back from this change because they believe they don't have enough help or they fear that technicians will take over their jobs.

When we decided to have technicians start filling all prescriptions, we were determined to stick with that approach at all costs until we'd established a smooth routine. So during the transition, if it meant the pharmacist had to run the cash register or computer to keep him or herself up front, away from the counting station, that's what we did. Admittedly, running the cash register is no more glamorous than filling bottles, but taking on such a function may be the first step to getting out from behind the counter.

Do *something* different to break out of your traditional duties and change your comfort zone. It's okay if the first approach you try is not the ultimate solution. Continue to experiment with anything other than what you were doing previously. We tried all kinds of things to avoid picking up that spatula, such as putting away prescription bottles and bagging completed prescriptions. In this way, we became available for what we *really* should be doing—consulting with patients about their medications and health-related questions.

I was told by one chain executive, "If I see you behind the counter filling prescriptions, I'm going to give you a spatulectomy!" I don't know what a spatulectomy is, but I don't think I want one.

Solicit your staff's ideas about how systems can be altered to allow the pharmacist to spend more time up front with patients. Make sure you explain that this will take a greater effort on their part, but the rewards for them include more responsibility and satisfaction, as well as higher pay in many cases—especially if they earn national technician certification. It might seem to them at first like they are doing "your" work in addition to their own, but if you clearly present the rationale and benefits, they will buy in to the changes.

The ultimate goal is to create a work environment where pharmacists are responsible only for checking prescriptions, performing other functions required by law, and handling professional responsibilities related to monitoring and improving patients' drug therapy.

Once you've succeeded in getting pharmacists away from counting and pouring, it should be easier to convince management how costly it is to have a pharmacist doing technical functions. Conversely if you are the manager, you will be better equipped to add a technician as your prescription volume grows, rather than another pharmacist who has to count pills. This way, pharmacists can use their six or more years of education more effectively in the pharmacy—and in the health care system as a whole.

A Catalyst for Change

Try this strategy in your next staff meeting. Together, make a list of pharmacists' functions (those that the law requires pharmacists to do) and technicians' functions (everything else). Next, brainstorm about the barriers preventing pharmacists from the patient-oriented care they would like to spend more time on. Most of the barriers listed are likely to be technical functions that eat up pharmacists' time.

Next, discuss technicians' future roles, and your desire to get them started in that direction now, so that pharmacists can realize their own professional vision. You could talk about such topics as technician certification, the differences between a career and a job, and so on. This exercise is a great catalyst for eliminating technical functions from the pharmacists' plate and getting technicians pumped up about changing their duties.

Idea #52 Create a separate pharmacist "check station."

SEE RELATED IDEA #51

We had just remodeled our pharmacy, so we knew we couldn't make big design changes anytime soon, but we wanted to add a station where pharmacists could check prescriptions prepared by technicians. Our prescription volume had increased and we'd gone from one long counter to two "island" filling areas. We decided to get creative and work with what we had. So we moved the pharmacist "check station" in between the two islands.

In this position, we have what we call a "golden triangle" workspace. Instead of running all over the place, we take just two steps to the phone and computer, and two steps to the patient consultation area.

If you have one long counter top, it's ideal to position your check station at one end, near a phone and consultation area. Do your very best to stay there; avoid getting trapped in the regular filling process if at all possible.

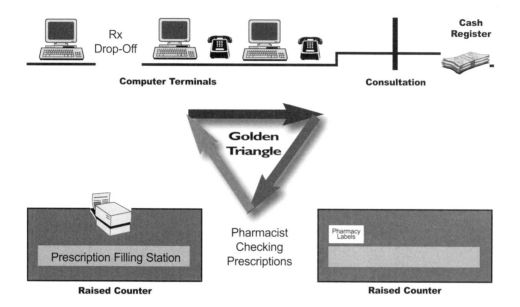

Rx Drop-Off

Computer Terminals

Consultation

Cash Register

Golden Triangle

Prescription Filling Station

Raised Counter

Pharmacist Checking Prescriptions

Pharmacy Labels

Raised Counter

If, like some pharmacists, you do not have adequate technician support, placing yourself in a position where you only check prescriptions, counsel patients, and telephone doctors may not work for you right now. If this is the case, I encourage you to experiment with doing things other than filling prescriptions—even some other nonprofessional task. It is very important that we get technicians to do all the filling. Pharmacists who are proficient on the computer, for example, could use this talent to prospectively monitor patient drug therapy. Having pharmacists run the computer is not a magical, catch-all solution, but it will allow you to experiment with an alternative workflow.

Idea #53 Use appointments for extended counseling sessions.

SEE RELATED IDEA #63, 91, 92, 100

Probably once a day or more, patients have complex questions that will take more time to address than you can give at the moment, and you would really like to help them. This presents you with an excellent opportunity to make an appointment with the patient.

For example, a patient who has just been diagnosed with asthma and has several questions comes in when you are very busy. You have a personal interest in helping patients with asthma, and would like to consult with the patient on peak flow meters and ways to reduce the chances of ending up in the emergency room with an asthma attack.

Decide upon a mutually agreeable time to schedule 15 or 20 minutes with the patient. Write the appointment time on the back of your professional business card (idea #92) and give it to the patient. Be sure to transfer the appointment time to your own calendar, as well.

You can meet in the pharmaceutical care work environment you've created in accordance with idea #91. It doesn't have to be anything fancy; just a semi-private place where you can provide a more in-depth consultation than is possible over the pharmacy counter.

You might even be surprised when the patient asks, "How much do I owe you?" Idea #100 discusses ways to pursue reimbursement for your professional services.

Idea #54 Reduce dispensing errors by using NDC codes.

We've never made a lot of errors in our pharmacy, but whenever we make one, it's distressing. Of course, everyone makes mistakes at one time or another, but prescription errors can have such grave consequences that we became determined to find a way to prevent them.

Our computerized prescription receipts include not only the quantity and price, but also the 11-digit National Drug Code (NDC) number on them. To reduce errors, a few years ago we started checking the codes on the receipts against the bottle we were filling the prescription from. It is only necessary to use the last six digits of the NDC.

Since our technicians do all the filling, pharmacists double check each prescription by comparing the NDC on the bottle with the

NDC on the receipt. There is a potential for error, however. If your technicians get in the habit of just copying the number as it is written on the receipt instead of taking it from the stock bottle, eventually the wrong drug goes into the vial you are filling for the patient. Be sure to emphasize this with them, or the system fails. It is absolutely critical that the NDC number be transferred in writing directly from the stock bottle to the prescription refill stub that the pharmacist is checking for accuracy.

Another potential glitch occurs when you are using a temporary, substitute product with a different NDC than the product that is active in your computer. Obviously, the best way to fix this is to change the NDC in the computer to reflect the stock bottle you are currently using.

As a general safety policy, technicians should be instructed to show the pharmacist each prescription they are filling for which the NDC doesn't match what they think is the right drug. Then have them change the NDC in the computer so that you are dispensing exactly what you are billing for.

CHAPTER 8

"If you don't like something,

change it. If you can't change it,

change your attitude."

—Maya Angelou

Third Party Issues

 Idea #55 Design a third party brochure.

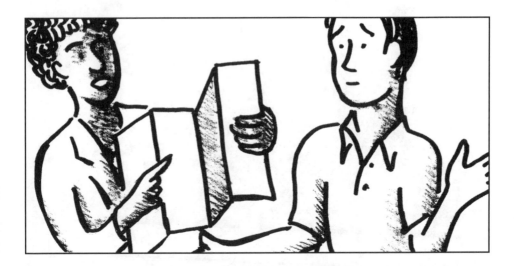

Most patients don't understand how third party insurance works. Insurance is confusing and complicated. Typically, patients know only that they pay insurance premiums—and thus they expect a service. Some pharmacies have developed a third party brochure to help their patients with this problem. Providing such a brochure to patients equips them to solve problems and knowledgeably address issues with their insurance company. Here's a starter list of what you might include:

- A definition of terms, such as "pharmacy benefits manager" and "generic equivalent."
- How medical insurance differs from prescription drug insurance.
- Why it's important to keep your drug card with you at all times.
- What a formulary is and how it is used.
- Why prescription claims are sometimes rejected by the insurance company and what to do when they are.
- How prescription claims are transmitted to the insurance company.
- Why your prescription drug card might change even though you have not changed employers or health care insurance providers.

The alternative to educating patients about how insurance works is to keep doing everything for them, and to take the blame for problems when they arise. Separate yourself from the third party, and your morale will improve. In addition, patients will see you as more of a friend than foe.

Idea #56 Be savvy when communicating third party rejection.

SEE RELATED IDEA #18, 43

When a procedure done in a doctor's office isn't covered by the patient's insurance, it's between the patient and his or her insurance company. Usually, billing for medical services takes place after the services are rendered. It's not until days or weeks after a medical checkup or procedure that the patient learns what was covered by insurance and what wasn't. But prescription coverage is determined online before the patient settles up with the cashier and exits the pharmacy. Therefore, patients automatically associate prescription claim rejections with the pharmacy.

Third party rejection is very difficult for some patients to accept. If they become irate and are unreceptive to your explanation of what happened, then stop. They now see the situation as "unfair," and you must keep that in mind. Anything you can say or do to let patients know you see the situation from their perspective will keep tension to a minimum. Neither reasoning with them nor displaying your knowledge of the third party policy will put you where you want to be.

If you've studied martial arts, you know that each type has different styles and techniques. Tae kwon do uses a forceful, aggressive approach; one punch or kick to the attacker, and the fight is over. In a similar vein, a quick, one-line explanation is acceptable to some patients. Tai chi practitioners deflect the aggressor to avoid injury to both themselves and their opponent. Employ a variation of this concept when the patient sees the situation as unfair. After you have deflected the patient's anger away from you by listening and empathizing with the patient about this unfair situation, you can focus on solving the problem together.

The best way to deal with patients facing a third party rejection is idea #18: "Here's what we can do." Before patients have time to get angry with you, start giving them choices. For example, if a prescription claim comes back indicating that the patient is not covered, try saying this: "Mrs. Jones, we're having difficulty processing your prescription claim today. Would you like to contact your employer, or would you prefer to pay cash?" Because you are giving Mrs. Jones instant choices, she doesn't have much time to become angry with you.

If it's possible that the problem is simple enough to be resolved on the spot, you can get patients involved by handing them the telephone right in the pharmacy immediately after you dial it (idea #43). As long as you empathize with patients, you are their ally, and you can continue about your work as they hold for their insurance company.

Another effective option is to say, "I could fill the prescription for a two- or three-days' supply, and if you get the problem resolved, just come in and we will rerun the prescription on your insurance card." This solution means the patient faces the minor inconvenience of another trip to see you. However, they don't usually mind because they're so happy that you have helped them. And the situation is likely to involve another trip to the pharmacy anyway, especially if the insurance company hasn't activated the patient in its system.

There are no hard-and-fast approaches to easing third party rejections, but a few good options are offering immediate choices, saying "here's what we can do," and offering patients your phone so they can solve the problem on the spot.

I know this may be hard for some pharmacists and technicians to believe, but when we use this approach, most people express their gratitude for all we have done for them before they leave the pharmacy. The old saying "less is more" is certainly true here.

Idea #57 Argue on behalf of the patient, and win.

SEE RELATED IDEA #42, 43

I don't think there's a better way to show patients you really care about them than to argue on their behalf while they listen, especially when you think their insurance company has treated them unfairly.

"I feel like a needle in a haystack," one of our patients told us, referring to her insurance plan. "You just can't get anywhere with them." Sometimes the expertise of a pharmacist is helpful in cutting through the bureaucracy, conveying salient information, and identifying alternative solutions to the patient's problem.

If you don't get anywhere with the person at the insurance help desk, ask to speak to the supervisor. Never threaten, use profanity, or raise your voice. Tell whoever you are speaking with that you appreciate their assistance and know they have done everything they can. If their supervisor is not available, request the supervisor's direct phone number. Alternatively, leave your name and phone number and ask that the supervisor call you back.

A different—but equally valid—time to argue on behalf of patients is when you know exactly why their coverage is being denied, but they won't accept any explanation in the book. And there's absolutely nothing you can do about it. So you make a 180-degree turn and model their behavior as closely as possible.

Imagine that a mother is picking up a prescription for her 19-year-old son, who is leaving for college. The claim is rejected by the insurance company with this statement: "Coverage is no longer in effect." You know that this patient exceeds the age limit for dependent coverage, but the mother becomes hostile and refuses to accept your explanation. As soon as you recognize that the mother is upset, change your approach. Forget what you know about the prescription plan, call the company, and argue on behalf of the patient. Do this even though you know the claim will be denied.

With the mother standing right next to you, speak to the insurance company in a serious, cordial tone. Repeat things that she just told you, such as, "They paid their premiums and I know they are supposed to have coverage. I don't understand why this is happening. They really need this medication." And so on. When you have run out of responses and the patient has come around to see you as the "good guy" trying to help, close the call. Tell the insurance company, "Well, this doesn't seem fair, and it doesn't make much sense to me. Would you please explain it to the patient? She is standing right next to me." Then, hand her the phone.

When we use this tactic in our pharmacy, we have found that even if the patient walks away angry after speaking with the insurance company, we get a "thank you" instead of a @#$!

Remember, while you're on the phone with the insurance company, the patient should be in earshot of you saying things like, "This isn't fair," "They need this medication," "It's very expensive," "They paid their premiums," "They haven't changed jobs in twenty years," and anything else you heard the patient say earlier. The grand finale: "I just don't understand this, the patient is standing right here, will you please explain it directly?" Then hand the patient the phone.

We have changed more patients' attitudes with this strategy than any other. They leave knowing that you exhausted all your efforts, and you know that you've taken control of a potentially hostile experience.

 ### Idea #58 *Communicate back to the insurance company.*

There are so many different prescription drug cards in use today that all kinds of problems can arise. Sometimes cards are missing a group number or you can't determine the subscriber number.

Maybe person codes are omitted or the name of the insurance company is not on the card. The American Pharmaceutical Association is working to establish a standardized card for pharmacy benefits management (PBM) companies, but in the meantime, pharmacists and technicians can help.

Seize every opportunity to inform the PBM or plan sponsor of the problems you are having, and suggest to patients that they tell their employer about problems.

It's not enough to simply express to the company what you think. You need to file a complaint. Call the company issuing the card and ask for customer service. If possible, speak to a supervisor. Tell him or her that the problem you are calling about is persistent and it is taking up a lot of your time. Ask what procedure you should follow to file a formal complaint.

If no supervisor is available, request that your information be forwarded to the person in charge, or ask for the name and phone number of whoever is in a position to make a difference. Write the person a short letter or e-mail, or leave a voice mail message.

Most insurance companies aren't really aware that prescription drug cards are a problem. I heard the CEO of a major PBM tell an audience of pharmacists that when his company's help desk is busy, the company assumes it is doing a good job of resolving problems for patients and pharmacists. Unless we tell such companies exactly what problems we are facing with prescription drug cards and other matters, and suggest ways to resolve these problems, they are unlikely to be addressed anytime soon. By calling and providing feedback, we are helping to bring insurance companies' attention to problems they are unaware of.

Idea #59 Have a sample on hand of a "good" insurance card.

The worst thing about nonstandard prescription drug cards is that they create delays for your patients, because all the information necessary to process the claim is not on the card. As a solution, we photocopied a good prescription drug card and

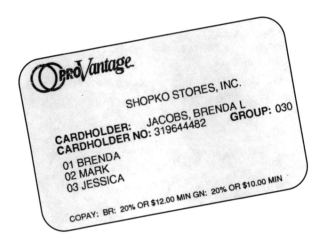

highlighted all the necessary information. For privacy, we whited out the patient's name and numbers. Now, when a patient's prescriptions are held up because their card has incomplete data, we give them a copy of a good card so they can see what information it is supposed to carry.

If you do this, show patients the specific differences between their card and your sample. Allow them to take the sheet of paper back to their benefits administrator. Better yet, ask who their benefits administrator is and get the phone number, so you can call yourself. Although in most cases you want to get patients to clear up insurance problems themselves, you may have more success than they will explaining to the benefits administrator why all their employees are having difficulty with prescription cards. When benefits administrators receive complaints and contact the insurance company or PBM on behalf of its employees, they are listened to because they influence whether the insurance plan is renewed. A complaint from someone representing a group of subscribers is far more powerful than one from a single individual.

Free Brochure

The American Pharmaceutical Association has developed a useful brochure about the problem of nonstandard prescription drug cards, which is available to give to your patients. It's called, "Have You Ever Wondered Why It Sometimes Takes Longer to Get Your Prescription Medicine?" and it contains an example of the information a prescription card should contain. The brochure may be downloaded for free from the APhA website (www.aphanet.org/stat/dcbrochure.pdf).

Idea #60 Have patients pay cash when they forget their prescription cards.

When patients who are new to the pharmacy come in without their prescription cards, pharmacists and technicians spend a lot of time investigating which insurance company to bill. This holds up everyone else waiting for their prescription. Maybe it's time to adopt a new policy.

It's not a problem when repeat patients forget their cards, of course, because the pharmacy has the cards on file electronically. But when new patients presenting a prescription order do not have their insurance cards with them, the best way to get them is to try calling another pharmacy that has their insurance information. If that effort fails, however, offer them their prescriptions for cash. Tell them they can return with their insurance card within three days for a refund.

When financial hardship is a concern, you can offer patients a few days' supply of medication for cash. Then reprocess the entire amount when they return with their card. Better yet, if you feel comfortable doing so, give them a couple days' worth of medication at no charge. This avoids long delays in your workflow while you search for information the patient is required to have to obtain prescriptions that are covered by insurance. Our objective is to help the most people with the least amount of disruption.

Idea #61 Reduce your risk of an audit.

Have you ever been audited by an insurance company? If not, it's just a matter of time before you are. According to H. Edward Heckman, president of the Pharmacy Audit Assistance Service (PAAS), the three primary reasons for financial retraction on an audit are:

- Missing signature logs.
- Insufficient documentation on "dispense as written" (DAW) prescriptions.
- Dispensing an incorrect days' supply.

Heckman says, "Poor maintenance of signature logs is the largest single source of audit problems and recoupment. Signature logs should be neatly filed chronologically into labeled notebook binders. If your pharmacy delivers or ships prescriptions, you will still need to maintain proof of delivery of services. Send signature logs on deliveries or keep accurate records of all shipments and deliveries."

Heckman says that missing signature logs are the largest revenue source from third party audits, and DAW codes come in a close second.

"The catch with DAW codes," he continues, "is that most third parties do not give pharmacies a second chance after the audit to verify missing information." Writing "dispense as written" in pen on the prescription hard copy is the key to minimizing this type of loss. It's important to transmit the correct DAW code on all prescriptions.

Finally, the proper days' supply must be transmitted to the insurance company, according to the prescriber's directions. "If the physician changes the directions, then create a new prescription," Heckman advises. "Be EXACT when you transmit the number of days' supply. If a prescription is written #100 taken TID, the correct days' supply is 33, not 30. Submitting an incorrect days' supply will cost you in an audit situation."

Heckman says you must always fill and bill a prescription exactly as it was written. "Many problems are averted by filling and billing the prescription as the doctor has written it. Approved changes are best handled by generating a new prescription order. Different information on the same prescription is a major audit flag."

Help With Audits

For assistance with pharmacy audits, you can call the Pharmacy Audit Assistance Service (PAAS), a national consulting firm that offers pre-audit planning and post-audit assistance to help reduce the cost of infractions. The service also analyzes third party contracts for language that places pharmacies in a compromising position and offers information to reduce your risk of an audit. You must be a member to take advantage of PAAS's services. Call 1-888-870-PAAS toll free for membership information.

$\widehat{\text{C}}$HAPTER 9

"Great spirits have

always encountered violent opposition

from mediocre minds."

—*Albert Einstein*

The Telephone
and Cash Register

 Idea #62 Have technicians answer all phone calls.

In a physician's office, the doctor never answers the phone. One doctor proudly told me, "Patients must be screened by the receptionist, and then the nurse, before they get to me." With today's increased emphasis on technicians, pharmacy has the opportunity to employ a time-management technique that physicians have benefited from for many years.

When nurses and receptionists screen calls for doctors, they gather pertinent data to help doctors make the most of their time. Technicians can screen pharmacists' calls for maximum efficiency, too. Here are some suggestions of ways they can do this:

- **Prescription transfers.** When another pharmacy calls to request that a patient's prescription be transferred, technicians should ask the caller for the prescription number, patient name, pharmacy name and phone number, and pharmacist's name. Then, after pulling the prescription hard copy for the pharmacist (if necessary) and bringing the prescription up on the computer screen, the technician can pass the telephone receiver to the pharmacist to authorize the transfer.

- **Questions from patients.** When patients call our pharmacy with a question, a technician obtains the patient name, prescription number (if applicable), and brief details about their question—just as a nurse conducts a preliminary assessment before doctors see patients. The technician writes the information on a slip of paper and hands it to the pharmacist, and also brings the patient's file up on the computer screen. If the answer is brief, the pharmacist may relay it back through the technician, but otherwise the pharmacist takes the phone and talks to the patient. I enjoy speaking directly to patients when my time allows, and I'm sure other pharmacists do, too.

If the technician tells us the patient needs to speak with a pharmacist, and the patient proceeds to request a refill, it's an opportunity to condition the patient not to use our time for this purpose. We kindly inform patients that we will transfer them back to the technician to process their order.

When technicians are busy, you may think it's easier to go ahead and take the prescription order yourself. But remember: If you always do what you always did, you will always do what you have always done. Nothing will change.

Idea #63 Call patients back later with responses.

Occasionally, pharmacists are too busy to take phone calls other than new prescriptions. When this situation arises—often around 5:00 pm—our technicians obtain the patient name, phone number, prescription number, and any other pertinent information. Then they state that the pharmacist will call back as soon as possible to give full attention to the patient's question.

If the patient has a simple "yes or no" question, the technician will relay the information to pharmacist without interrupting workflow. The pharmacist can give a quick response and avoid taking the call altogether. Nurses relay messages to patients from doctors all the time—why shouldn't technicians do the same for us?

When patients have complex health concerns, consider scheduling an appointment (idea #53). The patient will benefit from your expertise and you will gain loyalty by showing how much you care.

Idea #64 Answer "No" to "Can you hold, please?"

SEE
RELATED
IDEA
#81, 82

How often have you called a doctor's office only to hear, "Can you hold, please?" Tiring of this common occurrence with one clinic in particular, I decided to try something different. The next time I called and was asked, "Can you hold, please?" I said, "No, I'm sorry. This is Mark, the pharmacist next door. Can you put me through to Dr. Jones or his nurse, please?"

"Okay," the receptionist replied, "just one moment." And the rest is history.

In the past I always said, "Sure, I'll hold," and then I waited patiently. The very day I decided to try a different approach, however, I got a different response. Now I always use some variation of this approach.

Next time you are asked to hold when trying to reach a physician, say something like: "I'm sorry, I really can't. This is John at Hometown Pharmacy, and I need to speak with Dr. Jones's nurse to clarify a prescription received today. Could you please transfer me?" The receptionist will probably say, "Sure, no problem."

Idea #81 gives specific tips for accelerating right past the receptionist to get through to the doctor. For the ultimate solution to being placed on hold, obtain direct phone numbers to the doctor or the nurses' station, as outlined in idea #82.

Idea #65 Never be on hold for more than two minutes.

SEE
RELATED
IDEA
#43

Yeah, right! Next to impossible, unless you decide to enforce a two-minute limit yourself. If you are put on hold and two minutes elapse, you can either hang up, or—if the call involves a third party problem—give the patient the phone.

If you hang up, call the number right back. Explain that you have already been on hold and that you are pressed for time. Think about it: If you were calling a physician, and the situation were reversed, there's no way the physician would waste his or her time on hold for a pharmacist.

"Pharmacists are passive," lamented a group of pharmacists at a conference I attended. "They are way too nice." We agreed that we have to decide what we want, and accept nothing less. It's not necessary to be rude to get what you want. Know what results you're seeking and be firm, direct, and cordial.

Idea #66 *Urge patients to use voice mail for refills.*

Voice mail and answering machines are excellent tools for receiving phone-in prescription refills. In an established pharmacy, anywhere from 20 to 80 prescription orders can be in the fill queue when you arrive in the morning, waiting to be completed before the store opens. Actively promoting the use of voice mail and answering machines reduces the number of phone calls you have to take directly. As a result, you reduce the number of patients who expect "on demand" service, you spread your workload more evenly throughout the day, and you can focus on emptying the fill queue with less pressure.

Of course, a few patients still have rotary phones and thus can't make use of pushbutton features. Others refuse to use the latest technology or find it too confusing. But the rest are all yours, ready to be conditioned to use the telephone for ordering their refills in advance.

Our company prepared an informational letter for us to include with all new and refill prescriptions telling patients that voice mail is now available for refill requests. The letter explained that the voice mail service would benefit them by saving time. After distributing the letters for a few months, we stopped giving them to everyone, but we still keep a supply near our printer and use them daily for new patients and for others who bring in their prescription bottles rather than calling in refills. When these patients pick up their prescriptions, we explain that we are including some "good information about receiving faster prescription refill service by using our voice mail system."

Touch Tone Refill System

Getting your refills is as easy as 1, 2, 3.

Step 1: Enter **1** to access the Touch Tone System.

Step 2: Enter the number referring to the **time** you plan on picking up your prescription or enter * to pick up your prescription tomorrow.

Step 3: Enter your **7-digit prescription number**, wait for the automated voice to repeat it back, then press 1.

We often conclude counseling sessions by telling patients how simple our voice mail is to use. We also inform them that if they have difficulty with voice mail they can still call ahead and save themselves (and us) time. When patients tell us they have a rotary phone or are uncomfortable with new technology, we still emphasize the benefits of phoning ahead and assure them that it's easy to bypass the voice mail system when necessary. We also include a memo with their prescription telling them about the benefits of calling in their prescriptions in advance. It reads something like this:

Dear Patient,

Your time is very valuable to us. We can now offer prescription refills without the wait. Simply phone in your refill numbers 24 hours in advance and your prescription will be waiting for you the next day. This will allow us to help everyone more efficiently—particularly those patients who are feeling ill or have just been discharged from the hospital.

If you forget to call 24 hours in advance, we can still take a refill request for later on in the same day.

Thank You.

At my bank, there's a sign saying "Please have your deposit slip filled out ahead of time . . . so we can give you our BEST SERVICE." When I first read it, I thought to myself, what a polite way to say "Don't waste our time by filling out your deposit or withdrawal slip at the teller window." In the same vein, our letters and reminders condition patients to use our time wisely.

Idea #67 When you must, use the last resort.

I hesitated to include this idea, because it will make every manager and supervisor in the country cringe. The last resort for handling the phones is to place all lines on hold.

Everyone who has worked in a busy pharmacy has, at one time or another, been so overwhelmed that there seems to be no way out. Maybe your lead technician called in sick, another is on break, you need to phone doctors about three different prescriptions, two prescriptions need to be reprocessed because the patient's insurance information changed and they didn't give you the new card beforehand. The prescription wait time has gradually increased to 30 minutes, your patients are not happy, and everyone's patience is growing thin. All of this creates a very stressful situation.

There are many ways to manage telephones and workflow other than putting all lines on hold—and the strategies described in this book are among them. But sometimes, you must go for the last resort.

Because of all the efficiencies we've built into our practice, we haven't used the last resort for at least five years. Before that, we put all lines on hold maybe once or twice a year, for a maximum of 10 minutes. And each time we did it, we were beyond busy by anyone's definition. We were deluged and the situation was out of our control.

If you incorporate the ideas in this book, you should be able to manage your workflow so you can avoid the last resort. In all honesty, if you need to use idea #67, you probably don't have enough support staff or there is a flaw in your pharmacy's operating procedures.

Idea #68 Don't let pharmacists run the cash register.

As long as you always have at least one other employee working with you, you may find this idea helpful for freeing pharmacists' time for professional responsibilities.

For us, finding a way to get pharmacists off the cash register was a struggle. Since we were up at the window anyway, counseling patients picking up prescriptions, it seemed natural to stay there and ring up purchases. We'd try calling the cashier over from behind the counter, where he or she was busy doubling as a counting technician, but more often than not, the pharmacist got stuck running the cash register.

Then our store bought new cash registers. Everyone was told to sign up for a time to be trained to run them. We were midway through training the technicians when it occurred to me: If pharmacists don't go through the training, they won't know how to run the register. If they don't know how to run the register, they will no longer feel compelled to do it. Yes, this meant more work initially for our technicians, but they have incorporated it into their daily regime. They know that ringing up purchases is no longer a task that the pharmacists handle.

Maybe you feel you are not quite ready to take pharmacists off the registers. But think about how our friends in hospital pharmacies and the mail order business operate: Pharmacists do not ring up purchases there. Furthermore, pharmacists are very expensive cashiers!

Idea #69 Have patients take all purchases up front.

SEE
RELATED
IDEA
#68, 74

We used to let patients take their prescriptions to a register in the front of the store, along with their other purchases, simply to give them the convenience of writing only one check or doing only one transaction. That way they could pay for their prescription, hair gel, toilet paper, and greeting cards all at one time. Then we realized that allowing patients to take purchases elsewhere lets the pharmacy focus on filling prescriptions and counseling patients. Now we encourage patients to use the front register—even if all they have to pay for is a prescription.

Of course, when patients have a few small items to buy, there's nothing wrong with ringing them up in the pharmacy . . . unless it interferes with the service you provide to other patrons. One pharmacy I know of used to have a cashier who would ring up an entire cart full of merchandise while other people waited to get their one prescription and leave. Service was often compromised for several patients while providing a convenience for one. That makes no sense at all.

Idea #70 *Remove one or both registers.*

Our pharmacy has two consultation windows, each with space for a cash register. Because we allow patients to take prescriptions to a register at the front of our store, it struck us as logical to remove one of the pharmacy registers. This way, at one window we could quickly counsel patients who are in a hurry and want to pay up front. We never had enough help to run both registers, anyway.

Granted, some pharmacies have multi-talented cashiers who can do two things at once, but you rarely go into a department store and see someone working two registers. When customers come to you they deserve your undivided attention, and you can't give it if you're operating two pieces of equipment. Expecting one person to run two registers means giving bad service and stealing time from other tasks such as bagging completed prescriptions and putting drugs away.

After getting rid of one cash register, the next step is to remove them all from the pharmacy. (An exception would be if you must handle transactions at a drive-up window.) Although some pharmacies have tried this and failed, I believe that removing all registers could be successful if tested in a pharmacy ready to elevate its practice to the next level. With no purchases to ring up, pharmacists and technicians could dedicate themselves to consulting and accurately dispensing prescriptions. Furthermore, pharmacists could expand their services to include disease state management and health screening.

Idea #71 *If the store has other registers, limit the operating hours of the pharmacy's register.*

A while ago, faced with tight payrolls and limited availability of technicians, we were forced to experiment with the hours our cash register operated. We found we were able to close it the first and last hours of each day—and thus we shaved 40 hours per month from our payroll budget.

We communicated the shortened register hours to our patients in a positive, professional manner.

"Our register is not open yet" or "Our cashier hasn't arrived yet this morning," we'd politely tell them. Alternatively, we'd explain that the register would open at 9:00 am (an hour after the pharmacy opened). A sign in the consultation area, near the register, read: "This register is closed. You may pay for your prescriptions at another register."

Initially this was an experiment. We wanted to see if we could shorten our register hours without causing major disruptions or decreasing the level of service. Communicating with our supervisor to reassure him that we could still provide excellent service while using our payroll more effectively, and coordinating our efforts with the main store manager were critical to our success. We continued with this strategy for several months, until our payroll eased up and we could afford more staff.

An advantage we gained from reduced cash register hours was fewer interruptions, which allowed us to process more prescriptions from voice mail early in the morning and to perform our end-of-day closing procedures on time. We discovered it's a great tool when resources are tight—and it may be a way to ease into removing the pharmacy's cash register.

Idea #72 *Limit the number of items you accept at the register.*

We experimented with a sign near the cash register that said, "Please limit your pharmacy purchases to 6 items or less." A few people with eight or nine items would push the limit, but as a general rule we prevented people from ringing out more than 10 items in the pharmacy.

We didn't need to leave the sign at the register for more than a few months before patients started voluntarily requesting to take their purchases to another register. They were conditioned to enhance the efficiency of service by paying for their prescriptions at another register whenever they had other purchases. Eventually we took

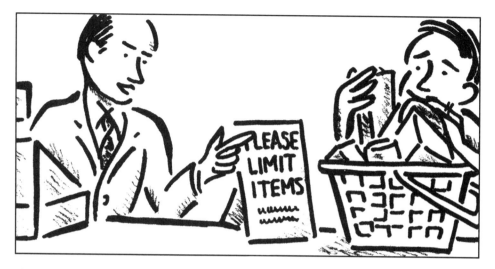

the sign down, and now it's the norm for patients with multiple purchases to use another register. It's difficult to imagine that it used to be any other way.

Idea #73 Limit the types of items you accept at the register.

After successfully limiting the number of items patients could ring out in the pharmacy, we decided to restrict the types of merchandise we would allow. We wanted to focus our efforts on providing the best service we could to patients with prescription and over-the-counter medications to purchase.

First we retrained customers buying clothing, toys, household furnishings, automotive products, and the like by telling them that we couldn't accept those items at the pharmacy register anymore. If they asked why, we explained that ringing up purchases was hindering our ability to help patients with their medication needs and health care questions. Nothing beats honesty!

Next we focused on eliminating smaller items like videos and greeting cards. The problem wasn't only how long it took to ring up a few small items, but also the time-sapping business of dealing with price discrepancies or sale items. After people became aware that we were not equipped to ring up their entire cart, we loosened up a bit.

We always ask patients, "Would you like to pay for your prescription up front with your other items?" We used to give them choices—pay here or up front—but found that by eliminating the offer to ring up the purchases in the pharmacy, patients are more inclined to take them up front.

Idea #74 *Use bar codes and magnetic tracking systems.*

Here's a nifty idea if you're concerned about theft of prescriptions to be paid for at another register. Try placing on prescriptions the same magnetic, anti-theft tags often used on compact disks and videotapes. You can attach them to the paper prescription receipt or actually affix one to each prescription vial, and put the vial inside a clear plastic bag that you hand to the patient. Check into getting smaller tags if the ones used elsewhere in your store are too large for a prescription container.

It's always possible that patients can tear them off, but the same potential exists with CDs, videos, diabetes test strips, and all kinds of merchandise. As long as your store security manager is involved in the process, you have an excellent resource for minimizing loss.

If your store is in a high-theft area, consider allowing only prescriptions costing less than $10 to be paid for outside the pharmacy. You could also track the prescription numbers that are going to the front registers by filling in a log at the pharmacy consultation window and having another up front for the cashiers to fill in. Each night, the logs can be compared at closing. You can contact patients by phone or letter if a missing entry suggests they didn't pay.

Some pharmacies have an electronic bar code number assigned to each prescription by their computer software. If your system doesn't currently use this technology, it might be time to look into it. The principle is similar to that used by overnight shipping companies, such as Fed Ex. Each item is given a unique tracking number readable by a bar code scanner. The item can be tracked by its bar code to determine its exact location.

In the prescription tracking system, each tracking number is removed from the system when the item is paid for at the cash register. At the end of each day, all remaining prescriptions—those that were not yet picked up—are scanned with a portable scanner. From the report generated, you can see which prescriptions were potentially not scanned or not paid for. Making courteous follow-up calls to the patients in question allows you to determine if they "forgot to pay for the prescription" or if a system processing error occurred.

Whichever system you choose—magnetic tags or bar codes—the result will be a more efficient pharmacy operation that allows you and your staff to focus on professional services.

CHAPTER 10

"The best time to plant a tree

was 20 years ago.

The second best time is now."

—Chinese Proverb

Doctors and Nurses

Idea #75 Train doctors and nurses to use voice mail and fax for prescriptions.

More and more, pharmacies are relying on fax machine and voice mail technology to streamline their pharmacy practices. Until electronic data transfer comes along, faxes and voice mail are useful tools for handling prescription refills when state law allows. Although we are sold on the ideas mentioned earlier about having patients handle their own prescription refills, I don't want to discourage the use of other effective prescription refill approaches if they work well in a particular location.

If you acquire a fax machine, for example, you can draft a letter to all major clinics in your area asking them to send all prescription orders by fax whenever possible. Before you mail it, tell each nurse and physician who gives you prescription orders that they will soon receive a letter informing them of your new fax machine. State in any oral or written communication the importance of including the three items in idea #76. Your level of success will be determined by your commitment and persistence with the doctors and nurses.

Some pharmacies offer voice mail technology to physicians and nurses for calling in new prescriptions and renewals. This useful time management tool allows pharmacists to retrieve new prescriptions at their convenience, when they're not busy helping patients. It is hoped that in the future, state boards of pharmacy will work to allow transmission of prescription data to pharmacies using e-mail or other forms of electronic technology.

Idea #76 Set information standards for nurses and physicians who phone in prescription orders.

How many times does a nurse or physician call in a prescription and say, "Renew so and so's HCTZ—they've had it there before," or, worst case scenario, "Refill all meds"? And later you discover that the patient has never gotten that prescription at your pharmacy before. Or the dosage was increased, so the patient is using more than the records indicate—and thus the insurance company rejects it as "refill too soon." An even more worrisome problem occurs when the patient continues to take the medication as before, based on instructions the pharmacy had on file, but the doctor had intended for the patient to increase or decrease the dose.

Setting standards for the information that prescribers give you helps ensure quality care for patients. If a doctor or nurse balks, explain that your company has changed its policy on phone-in prescriptions and you must collect standard information. Accept no less than the following on every prescription order that is phoned in by a doctor's office:

- Current drug strength
- Current directions
- Patient's date of birth

In some pharmacy markets, physicians and nurses do not provide pharmacists with an acceptable level of information about how the patient's medication is supposed to be taken. At your local pharmacy association meeting, consider discussing the issue of receiving standard details on phone-in prescriptions. If everyone in your geographic area bands together, it will make the task of improving the quality of care a lot easier. As a group, you can change the norm in your community.

Nurse Conversion

I once sent a bill to a nurse who had refused to give me current medication information when she phoned in a prescription refill. She assured me that she wanted the same medication to be prescribed as the last time, so we dispensed the medication based on our previous instructions.

Later, the patient returned with the medication, explaining it was wrong and insisting on a refund. I gave his money back and threw away the medication. Then I billed the nurse for $65.

"What's this?" the nurse asked when she called me the next day. I explained nicely that because she did not take the time to look at this patient's chart, he got the wrong medication. We had even questioned the patient carefully to verify that the medication was correct.

I paused. Then I said, "I'll tell you what. I won't bill you for the patient's medication this time, but I need the milligrams, directions for use, and date of birth for every single patient from now on." I explained that we dispensed incorrect prescriptions at least every other week because prescribers failed to give us current information. It was costing us over $1,000 a year, I emphasized, and worse yet, it could jeopardize a patient's safety. She apparently had no idea of the potentially severe consequences of her omission, and agreed to comply with our request.

Occasionally she leaves a voice mail message and forgets to include all the pertinent data for safe dispensing. We always call back and verify the most current information. It's amazing how quickly nurses decide to look up information when you say that you would like to take their name for documentation purposes, just in case there is a problem.

 Idea #77 Try three approaches when physicians want you to call them about prescription orders.

When patients need refills, some physicians tell them to call their pharmacist and have the pharmacist call the physician. This works out fine if, when you call the doctor's office, someone takes your call and gives you the prescription order within 60 seconds. But what about those situations in which you call and the staff at the physician's office has no idea what you are calling about? What about the times when it takes them five minutes to find the information? Here are three possible solutions:

1. Explain tactfully that your time is very valuable, and you don't mind calling them if they have the information ready. Seize this opportunity to explain that the process would be more efficient if they called the prescription order into your voice mail or faxed

it to you. Let them know that you will be happy to continue calling their office for prescriptions as long as they are able to make the process efficient for both of you. Tell them this every time you wait more than 60 seconds.

2. If you repeatedly explain to a physician's office how to improve the efficiency of the prescribing process, and it fails, start calling the patients back. Let them know that the doctor didn't have anything ready to phone in. Request that they try contacting their doctor to see if there is some kind of mistake. We did this with a clinic in our area, and after we made a few calls to patients, the clinic must have changed its procedures. Now it always has the prescription information ready to convey to us.

3. Fax the prescription request to the doctor's office. This is probably the best of all three ideas, because you don't have to wait on hold.

At our pharmacy, setting the standards we will accept and conditioning others to comply with them allow both patients and health care providers to get the most from our services.

Squelch Bad Habits

One physician in our area, after calling in a prescription to us, used to say, "Would you please call the patient at home and let her know I have called in the prescription for her?" My response: "Oh sure, and why don't you tell all your doctor friends about this, so we can call every patient when prescriptions are phoned in?" I'm just kidding! But can you imagine if we had let a bad habit like this take hold?

We always took the message and filled the prescription like any other order. We knew that if the patient wanted to call us to see if it was ready, he or she was free to do so. We left it at that.

Be careful not to encourage new habits among prescribers that you may regret. Your time is valuable, and if they don't see it that way, it's clear they haven't considered that your time is directly related to that of your patients and to the quality of service you can provide.

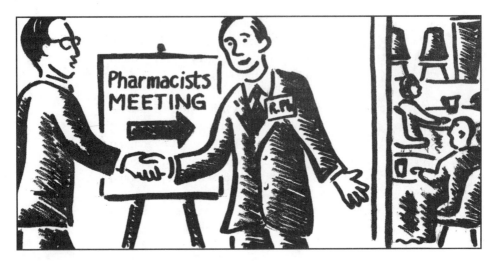

 Idea #78 Invite a physician to a local pharmacists' meeting.

Pharmacists and physicians take care of the same patients. Yet we have very little direct contact with each other. Interaction between health care professionals has tremendous merit. Imagine the possibilities that can result from inviting a different doctor to a local pharmacy meeting twice a year. You can bring in the physician as a speaker or simply as a guest, but the overall purpose is to have a dialogue about efficiency of patient care and ways to address issues central to both pharmacists and physicians.

Extend the invitation by calling the physician, and follow the call with a written confirmation or fax. The pharmacists who will be at the meeting should think through what they hope to accomplish and decide on the meeting's goals ahead of time. Some ideas for discussion will get better results than others. It would be courteous to give the doctor a list of topics beforehand so he or she knows what to expect. Some topics you might consider are how to handle prescription drug abusers or insurance issues affecting care.

To involve physicians in your local pharmacy meeting, you might also try these ideas:

- Have a drug company sponsor a continuing education program for both pharmacists and physicians.

- Extend to physicians an open invitation to any of your regularly scheduled meetings, to give them an opportunity to bring up concerns of their own.

You could also develop a list of pharmacists' concerns to talk about at the meeting. But remember, the physician may feel like the lone duck among the geese. Be careful not to intimidate or attack him or her personally.

A Lesson from EMTs' Education

I spent 11 years as a volunteer emergency medical technician (EMT), intermediate level, for a local ambulance service. Back in the early 1970s, when our nation's emergency medical system (EMS) started gaining sophistication, emergency room doctors grew concerned about what was happening in the field. They were not always pleased with the pre-hospital treatment being rendered and thus they became more active in the EMT training process. As a result, EMTs developed a better understanding of physicians' expectations about patient care. Today, patients can expect to receive top-notch medical care in areas serviced by advanced-level EMTs and paramedics because doctors got involved in setting standards and delivering training.

The way I see it, pharmacists are in the same situation as EMTs 20 years ago. If physicians were to provide input into what we tell their asthma and diabetes patients, they would feel more comfortable about our role in patient care. The sooner we include physicians in our efforts to expand services into the realm of pharmaceutical care, the sooner we reach our goal of a "seamless health care system."

Idea #79 Start asking for diagnosis codes or indications.

A few years ago, it was almost unheard of for a physician to share a diagnosis code. Now, with the advent of managed care, physicians have come to expect that they must provide more information to insurance companies before claims for patient care services will be paid. This is a plus for pharmacists, because now we have what physicians see as a "valid excuse" for requesting the diagnosis. When you are speaking to a doctor or nurse about a patient's drug therapy, start requesting a diagnosis code "for the insurance company."

If we don't know the indication a certain drug was prescribed for, it's very difficult to counsel a patient, and it's especially tough when the medication prescribed has many different indications. Conditioning other health care professionals to share relevant patient information enhances our ability to care for our patients.

Idea #80 *Stop apologizing to doctors and nurses.*

SEE RELATED IDEA #76

Do you ever find yourself calling a physician and saying, "I'm sorry for bothering you, but I have a concern about . . . ?" This wording sends a negative message to physicians because it suggests that we are, in fact, bothering them. Instead, begin by saying, "I have a concern about one of your patients." Such phrasing lets the physician know your call is both relevant and necessary for providing quality care to the patient.

Pharmacists interact with physicians daily. If we apologize to them every time we call, we plant the idea that we are somehow doing something wrong. Our concern is the safety and well-being of our patients—the same concern physicians have. Never apologize to a physician unless you truly mean to ask forgiveness for some wrongdoing.

Nurses, too, sometimes make us feel like we are pestering them for information. Remember how, in idea #76, we talked about the importance of receiving all of the necessary details for prescription orders? Push aside any feelings that you are being a bother. If we are persistent with our expectations, we can condition nurses to give us what we need.

One pharmacist I used to work with asked a nurse on the phone why she never provided complete prescription information. Her response was, "Because it's easier this way." He replied, "Easier for you, or easier for me?" She wasn't happy, but I'm sure he made an impression on her. We all work in a harried environment, he emphasized to her, but that gives us no reason to compromise the quality of care we provide.

Idea #81 Accelerate past the receptionist.

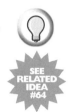

SEE RELATED IDEA #64

How can you accelerate past the gatekeeper to reach doctors or nurses directly? Receptionists serve as a center for routing messages, so if you must ask a question or clarify a medication order you have to navigate around them. Among ways to do this successfully:

- Get to know receptionists by name. If they mention their name, repeat it back to them with a greeting. People like to hear their own name.

- Once in a while, to establish rapport, ask them how their day is going.

- Make a point of saying hello to them if you visit that clinic for any reason. Delivering Christmas candy is a nice way to make an appearance at clinics you deal with—and a great opportunity to meet the receptionist in person.

- When you call with a question, explain to the receptionist that you just got off the phone with nurse so and so (assuming this is true) and that you need to clarify something quickly.

When you're frustrated with the way things are, try to change them! Don't accept the status quo. Physicians expect to speak directly to pharmacists, and pharmacists have a right to expect the same.

Take a Music Break

Sometimes a clinic has really cool jazz playing in the background when you're on hold waiting to speak to a doctor or nurse. Enjoy it! This book gives lots of tips for reducing your time spent on hold, but sometimes you need a mental break. There's nothing wrong with indulging in 60 seconds of your favorite music. Best of all, no one else knows you're on break!

Idea #82 When direct clinic phone lines are available, obtain the listings.

Obtain lists of direct phone numbers for the doctors' and nurses' stations at the major clinics you deal with. If you think creatively, you'll find it's not so hard to accomplish. We received just such a list by asking a prominent doctor to supply one (see box). You can also ask nurses how to go about getting phone lists, or even request their individual numbers, assuring them that you will use them only to phone about patients they have seen that day. (Questions about patients seen on other days are probably best dealt with through the receptionist, so the chart can be ordered and delivered to the nurses' station.)

How We Did It

In one of our local pharmacy association meetings, we were discussing ways that pharmacists and physicians could work more efficiently together. We complained about always having to go through a receptionist, just like the general public. If doctors have a direct phone line to pharmacists, we reasoned, they should reciprocate. After raising other concerns involving physicians, we decided it would be beneficial to invite a physician with some clout to one of our meetings.

That day, we first discussed things like insurance problems and non-AB rated generic medications before proposing our idea of having a list of phone numbers for doctors' and nurses' stations. We gave our rationale for needing them and guaranteed that we would only call for clarification of prescriptions they had just written. This would benefit physicians and nurses, we explained, because it would reduce paper phone messages and the need to call us back. He agreed it was a good idea, and three days later we had a whole list of phone numbers for every physician in the clinic. The list also included their fax numbers and their days off.

CHAPTER 11

"Get a good idea and stay with it.

Dog it, and work at it until it's done,

and done right."

—Walt Disney

Managing Your Time with Pharmaceutical Representatives

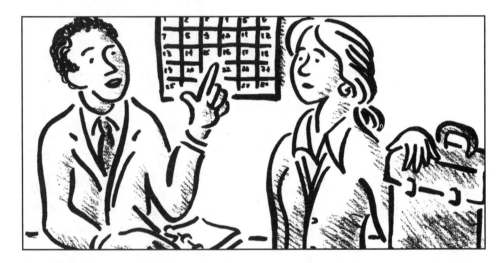

 Idea #83 Give pharmaceutical reps a time limit of one minute.

SEE RELATED IDEA #84, 88

You are the gatekeeper to your own time, but many pharmacists fail to control their time wisely. We can better manage our days using some simple techniques.

Pharmaceutical representatives sometimes eat up our time when we are busy. They come to see us without an appointment, interrupting our day. Our first priority must be patients who are waiting for their prescriptions or who have a question.

It is important, however, to receive detailed information about new products on the market, so meeting with reps can be worthwhile when you're able to squeeze it in. If you are very busy and decide to give the pharmaceutical representative some time, limit the visit to one minute. You might say, for example: "Hi, how are you today? As you can see, I'm very busy right now, so I can only listen for one minute. Please be brief." Most reps will respect your request.

When pharmaceutical representatives specialize in diseases for which you have decided to provide disease management services, you may want to give them extra time. If you can afford to commit a few more minutes on the spot, fine. A better approach, however, may be to tell the rep that you're very interested in what she has to say and would like to schedule an appointment so you can ask questions. Pharmaceutical representatives can be an excellent source of information, and their company may sometimes be willing to provide financial support for a disease state monitoring program or other idea you have.

Idea #84 Change your location when you speak with reps.

I read an article on time management that described a technique used by business executives. Each of their workdays is divided into increments, and they decide in advance how their time will be spent and how much they can allocate to each appointment. If a person wants to meet with the executive, he or she may be allotted 15 minutes. When the time is up, the executive gets up from the chair and starts walking to the door. The door opens, and hands are shaken. If the visitor doesn't leave right after that, the executive begins talking to the secretary or goes into another office. This is an effective way of signaling that the time is up. (Some executives might instead have their secretary call into their office and say, "It's time for your board meeting." Or, if they are meeting with an employee, they will go to the employee's office so they control the conversation's conclusion.)

Important to note in the example above is that the executive decided how much time to spend with the visitor, and when time was up, location was changed to signify that the conversation was over.

Pharmacists can use the same technique. Inform your staff in advance that from now on, you will handle drug rep meetings differently. The next time a rep comes to see you, change your location by walking several steps in front of the prescription area. In a chain department store, walk all the way to one of the aisles if possible.

When the amount of time you decided to allow has elapsed, use your walk-away power. Shake the rep's hand and thank her for coming, then leave.

Another option is to have a technician beckon you for a phone call or a consultation after a certain amount of time has passed.

Idea #85 Use the "stroll and nod" technique.

The "stroll and nod" technique is another way to signal to someone that your conversation is over. To do this, you start walking sideways, away from the person you are speaking with, while nodding in gratitude for the visit. You can initiate the stroll and nod with or without a handshake—whichever you feel most comfortable with at the time.

If you have already changed locations from your work station to the pharmacy floor or store aisle, this technique works well for letting you get back to business. If you are still in your pharmacy work station, take a restroom break as a signal that it's time for the visitor to leave, or simply thank the person for his or her time, and go about your work.

Idea #86 Give reps who drop in no time at all.

You don't want to sound rude, but your time is valuable. If you're too busy to see a pharmaceutical representative who drops in, diplomatically let him know that "it just isn't going to happen today" and thank him for coming. If possible, suggest a return visit tomorrow at a time when you know you are likely to be less busy or when another pharmacist's schedule overlaps with yours. Other alternatives:

- Have the rep leave marketing materials with your technician so you can look at them later.

- Ask for the rep's business card so you can call when it's convenient for you to talk.

- Make an appointment for a specific day and time when the rep can come back to speak with you—or schedule a telephone conversation.

Pharmaceutical reps have a job to do. Be kind to them. They can be your allies when it comes time to promote a pharmaceutical care service for your patients. If you really want to speak with them, be sure to let them know. It's also helpful to give them a look at your professional services area (idea #91) so they can visualize where you intend to provide pharmaceutical care.

Idea #87 Create a policy of seeing pharmaceutical reps by appointment only.

For a while, it seemed like pharmaceutical representatives were coming to see us every day. We decided to condition them (just as we had conditioned patients to assist us with prescription refills) by informing them that in three months we would start seeing them by appointment only.

Hometown Clinic, S.C.
Pharmaceutical Representative Policy

- All representatives will sign in and out of the clinic, and document the reason for their visit.
- The authorized representative for the day will be required to wear an identification badge.
- The representative of the day wearing the badge will be given priority by the physicians.
- All representatives dropping off samples to physicians are asked not to engage in conversation unless asked.
- Abuse to the above policy will result in a six-month suspension of appointments, and a letter will be directed to their employer reporting their unprofessional behavior.

Suddenly, they started to ask us when the best time to visit would be. They would even call ahead to schedule a more convenient time with us. Imagine how pleasantly surprised we were—someone was being considerate about our time!

Our policy is a slightly more liberal variation of one I witnessed in a local clinic. While visiting my own doctor, I noticed a note posted at the reception desk near the entrance of the building. The policy it conveys (see box on previous page) leaves no question as to how pharmaceutical reps are expected to conduct themselves.

The clinic also has a request book in which doctors stipulate for pharmaceutical reps the specific samples of medications they would like to receive. Have you ever considered asking a pharmaceutical representative for something you need?

 ## Idea #88 Ask them to show you the money!

A few years ago, our local pharmacy association decided to close the gap with area doctors by creating a pharmacist/physician newsletter. We considered faxing it to avoid printing and mailing costs, but decided that a letter on colored paper would be more likely to get read.

Our goal in producing the newsletter was to gradually help doctors understand that pharmacists are capable of assisting them with management of their patients. We also hoped to promote pharmacist-physician interaction. We covered such topics as basic formulary information, state Medicaid procedures, and the need for pharmacists to receive diagnosis codes. We let physicians know that we offer inhaler technique training, diabetes education, and blood glucose monitoring services. We also announced that we have patient compliance information in our pharmacy profiles that would be useful for treating their patients.

We could have paid for it ourselves, but instead we sought funding from a pharmaceutical representative. In our sales pitch to the rep, we explained that the newsletter would help move the pharmacy profession forward and, most important, would improve patient care.

Pharmaceutical reps have spending accounts at their discretion. Since they are always asking us, "What can I do to help you?" we decided to tell them. We had plenty of the usual free notepads and pens, which we appreciate, but this would have a more beneficial impact. And we felt good knowing that the money went to better use than taking a doctor golfing!

Pharmaceutical reps would probably love to help pharmacists get legitimate projects off the ground that have the potential to improve patient care. Ask to see a copy of their company's mission statement, and consider showing them yours. Write a proposal for funding a "diabetes day" project to screen people for the disease or for the purchase of a lipid monitoring system. Maybe they can even supply you with a copy of a successful grant proposal that you can use as a model.

One pharmaceutical company gave us funds to cover the cost of organizing and promoting two local asthma presentations. By charging attendees a small fee, the pharmacy earned enough money to purchase a $750 Vitalograph for monitoring inhaler technique. Other pharmacies have been given diabetes test strips for doing monitor training or diabetes data management printouts, as well as for indirect payment of newspaper and radio advertising costs related to a sponsored event. The financial support is there if you know how to ask for it. As in writing a grant proposal, the more you practice asking, the better you will become at it.

When your staff works very hard and you feel they deserve to be rewarded, try this. The next time a pharmaceutical rep asks you to help out by providing some prescription prices, ask if he or she would be willing to buy pizzas for your staff in exchange for your time. Pharmaceutical reps sponsor luncheons or refreshments at hospitals and clinics all the time as a way to expose nurses and doctors to their products. It's part of their advertising budget.

Another idea is to request financial support to allow your pharmacy technicians to attend a state pharmacy meeting. Or you could ask for some "scholarship money" to offset technicians' expenses for taking the national Pharmacy Technician Certification Examination. Considering the millions of dollars pharmaceutical companies spend on direct-to-consumer advertising, it wouldn't hurt them to show support for pharmacy technicians.

CHAPTER 12

"What you do, or dream you can do, begin it.

Boldness has genius, power and magic in it.

Only engage, and then the mind grows heated—

Begin it, and the work will be completed!"

—Goethe

Professionalism

The first 11 chapters of this book focus on ways that pharmacists and technicians can reduce stress on the job and create a more professional work environment. Chapter 12 is dedicated to small steps you can take to adapt and grow as the pharmacy profession moves further in the direction of pharmaceutical care.

Idea #89 Think in terms of features and benefits.

Any good salesman will tell customers about the features and benefits of the product he or she is selling. Pharmacists, too, must identify specifically what they are offering patients in order to justify charging for a service. How will the service you are providing benefit or improve the life of the person you are trying to sell it to?

Defining features and benefits is essential when you bill patients and insurance companies for your services. The very first time I decided to charge a fee, it was for conducting a diabetes monitor training session for a young man who was accompanied by his concerned mother. I explained the features of the monitor I wanted to sell them and presented some information about diabetes. I also identified ways that my professional expertise would benefit them if they were interested in having a personal consultation of 30 to 45 minutes. I explained that:

- They would learn how to do finger sticks less painfully.

- They would learn how to obtain more accurate blood sugar readings.

- They would gain a complete understanding of how to use the monitor.

- The information I would give them, combined with the data from the monitor, would give them better control over the son's diabetes and reduce the chances of such complications as blindness, kidney disease, and circulatory problems.

During our conversation I told them about our ability to print computerized reports from their monitor, which enhances their diabetes control even more. I described my advanced training in diabetes and noted that as a feature of my consultation I provide detailed information leaflets that I've created personally.

I pointed out that being diagnosed with diabetes and learning how to manage it is a scary process for some people. By spending a little extra time with me now, I emphasized, they would come away with a fuller understanding of diabetes and a better ability to control it.

The mother and son appeared to be thoroughly convinced of what I was telling them. The research I had done on "selling" the value of my services was paying off. Next came the most difficult part for me—telling them about my fee.

When I said that I would have to charge them for my time, I was more nervous than when I took my pharmacy boards. Quite honestly, I didn't even know what to ask for. I blurted out a figure, and waited. I expected to hear, "It sounds nice, but thank you anyway," or some other rejecting response. Instead, the mother said "Yes. When can we schedule an appointment?" I was elated.

The appointment for the consultation arrived. We spent more time together than I originally had anticipated. I felt like I was finally getting to put some of my diabetes training to use. We were sitting down in the consultation area I created. I was actually helping patients by giving them the information and tools necessary for managing a complicated disease.

When it was all over the mother thanked me. She told me how nice it was to have someone take the time to help them. As she reached into her purse to pay for the consultation, she attempted to give me a tip in addition to the fee I'd said I would charge her. After repeated attempts to refuse the tip, stating that it was company policy, I agreed to ring the additional amount into the register.

I couldn't believe that someone was actually trying to give me more than I had asked for. I learned two things that day. One, my service has value. And two, it's worth more than I charged for it.

I hope that the story of my first success inspires you as it *still* inspires me. Remember: If we continue to provide services for free, the services carry no perceived financial value. Think carefully about the features and benefits of your services and how you can best communicate them to patients.

Idea #90 Precept students and listen to their ideas about pharmaceutical care.

It always takes work and commitment to stay on top of the latest in any profession—but making the transition to pharmaceutical care is proving more challenging than many pharmacists are prepared for. Pharmacy students can be invaluable for coming up with ideas and plans to get the ball moving.

Precepting students who attend pharmacy schools in your region affords a wonderful opportunity to gain new perspectives and try out new approaches. Why don't you incorporate a pharmaceutical care plan into an internship or clerkship? People pay lots of money to consultants to help them establish and promote new services. Pharmacy students can do it for free.

One student helped us greatly when we were having a difficult time deciding how to promote our disease state management services. Knowing that our pharmacy student had to complete a special project during his rotation with us, we delegated to him the task of designing a service to screen for cholesterol and educate patients about its effects on heart disease. Part of his mission was to develop ways to promote the service, as well. Thanks to his studies he had current knowledge about lipid disorders, and he was eager to create a pharmaceutical care program that put his knowledge to use.

During your students' training and orientation phase, ask them, "What is your concept of the ideal pharmacy practice work environment?" Do this before students get acclimated to the way you currently practice. Choose an aspect of their ideal that would be beneficial in your practice, and encourage them to create a plan for implementing it. Think how much more valuable this project will be to your practice site than simply having students do exactly what you do.

The last time we had a pharmacy student, I conducted this little training exercise. I asked her to count 30 pills, put them in a bottle, and place a label on it. "Good," I said. "Now that you know how to do that, you shouldn't have to do it again unless there's an emergency!"

For information on becoming a preceptor, call the clerkship or intern coordinator at your nearest pharmacy school or pharmacy internship board.

Idea #91 Create a pharmaceutical care environment.

SEE
RELATED
IDEA
#53

Most pharmacies were not designed with patient care in mind. Even so, you can create an environment conducive to pharmaceutical care without actually remodeling your pharmacy. All it takes is some creative thought.

To establish a patient care area, place a table and some chairs in an area that, ideally, gives some degree of privacy. Some pharmacies put the patient care area off to the side of the prescription counter, in full view of the public; others have it behind the counter in a spot that is out of the normal prescription workflow.

It doesn't have to look like a clinic. Just create a space that allows you to conduct a semi-private training or consultation session, and try it out the next time someone wants to learn how to use a blood glucose meter or inhaler. See how it works, and make adjustments to the space as needed. Other items you might have in the patient care area are a blood pressure kit with stethoscope and literature about asthma, diabetes, and other diseases.

Idea #92 Create a business card or redesign the one you have.

SEE RELATED IDEA #53, 88, 96

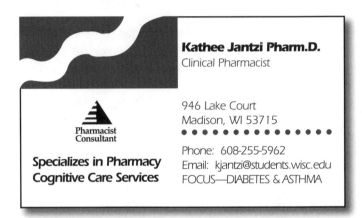

Kathee Jantzi Pharm.D.
Clinical Pharmacist

Pharmacist
Consultant

946 Lake Court
Madison, WI 53715
• • • • • • • • • • • • • •

**Specializes in Pharmacy
Cognitive Care Services**

Phone: 608-255-5962
Email: kjantzi@students.wisc.edu
FOCUS—DIABETES & ASTHMA

A business card is an excellent tool for coming across professionally and getting your name out to as many patients as possible. When patients receive your business card, it helps them associate your name with your face. You will no longer be just "the pharmacist," and it will be much more difficult for patients to become angry with you if they know you on a first-name basis.

The two keys to using business cards successfully are putting the right message on the card and distributing the card every chance you get.

Examples of messages you might include on your business card are, "Your medication experts," "We care about you," "Your health is important to us," or "Always here to answer your medication questions." Such messages add a personal touch and help patients understand that your primary concern is helping people, not putting pills in a bottle. You could also add such lines as "Clinical Pharmacist" or "Specializing in Diabetes Management" under your name to give patients an idea of your expertise. A good business card helps change patients' perceptions of who you are and what you do.

On your card, include your credentials after your name. This includes your college degrees as well as such designations as certified diabetes educator (CDE), Fellow of the American Society of Consultant Pharmacists (FASCP), Fellow of the American College of Apothecaries (FACA), and Board-Certified Pharmacotherapy

Specialist (BCPS). It's fine to use the acronyms on business cards rather than spelling out the full credential.

Not everyone achieves the credentials cited above, but many pharmacists complete certification programs in asthma, diabetes, smoking cessation, or immunizations. Put "certified in . . . " on your card to show that you have expanded knowledge in specialized areas.

Hand out your business card every time you recommend a product, calculate the dosage of an over-the-counter drug for a patient's infant, or consult with someone on a specific problem they are having. Always tell them that they should call you if they have any further questions or problems. Most people won't call, but the fact that you offered is worth its weight in gold.

Keep the cards readily available in your front shirt pocket, in the pocket of your slacks or skirt, or elsewhere on your person. A card is no good if you have to walk a distance to get it. When you're busy, you may forgo handing out your card in the interest of saving time. If your card is in your pocket, however, offering it to the patient takes only a second.

The more cards you give away the better chance you have of people getting to know you. Once they know you by name, the way they perceive you changes, and they are more likely to treat you with respect. When patients are frustrated or upset, they are less likely to refer to you as "this pharmacy" or "you people," and instead will interact with you in a more amicable way.

You can also give your business cards to pharmaceutical representatives who come into your pharmacy so they get acquainted with you and are more receptive to your requests for training materials or financial assistance (see idea #88). Finally, carry a handful with you when you go to association meetings. Such meetings present a great opportunity to network with other professionals, and business cards make it easy to exchange contact information.

Idea #93 *Post your credentials, certificates, and awards.*

SEE RELATED IDEA #14

Marketing your professionalism does not have to be limited to just one advertising medium. Handing out business cards is one way to market your professionalism; posting your credentials in plain view of patients is another. In hospital settings, patients tend to regard pharmacists as health care professionals, but put pharmacists in a retail store and the public's perception changes.

Most states already require that your license be posted in a conspicuous location. This same spot might be perfect for hanging other certificates or awards below each pharmacist's name. Good places for displaying framed credentials include your semi-private consultation area, the waiting area, or anywhere that is regularly in plain view of patients.

Pick out the nicest frames you can find, or have the framing done professionally. Some pharmacies post a photograph of the pharmacist with his or her background and the pharmacy's mission statement written immediately below it. Wisconsin offers a professional document signed by the governor for only $10.

You worked hard for your education. Display your credentials proudly. Once, a patient asked me if pharmacy is a two-year technical degree. I almost fell off my rocker! I began to wonder how many other people think that way. From that point on, I knew I had to communicate in any way possible that I am a health care professional who has passed a rigorous degree program and an intensive set of board exams.

Idea #94 *Support at least two pharmacy organizations.*

Most people who support the pharmacy profession see the value in the dollars they contribute to their state and national associations. I am continually perplexed, however, at the large numbers of pharmacists who do not become members of these organizations. Pharmacy, like many other professions, requires lifelong learning. For about the cost of one college credit per year, you can join an organization and reap the many benefits it offers.

In my own experience, pharmacists often don't join associations because their perception of value is too narrow. They believe that by spending $200, they should get $200 worth of product in return. They focus strictly on the journal they get in the mail—which costs maybe $45 a year—and think, "Big deal."

The fact is, associations work to serve the best interests of pharmacists and patients, and that's where a chunk of your dues payment goes. Associations are resource centers for pharmacists. They monitor key issues, provide solid information, and answer questions from members and the public. They offer high-quality continuing education, and through their annual and midyear meetings, they provide a forum where pharmacists can gather and exchange ideas.

Associations also lobby on behalf of legislation that favors pharmacists and their services, and they work to defeat proposed laws that could harm the pharmacy profession or the public. When a legislator or the press needs to know pharmacy's position on a specific area, they go to the association that professionally represents us. It costs money to maintain a building and professional staff, and that's also how some of your membership dollars are used.

If you're frustrated with workplace issues, voice your concerns to your state and national associations. "Laws don't pass automatically," said David B. Brushwood, J.D., a professor of pharmacy health care administration at the University of Florida, in a recent editorial. "It takes a lot of grassroots support for legislators to recognize that a bill is worthy of their support." He pointed out that pharmacists "are at least partially responsible for their own problems," and that they are "fully responsible for finding solutions." Too many pharmacists try to place the blame on boards of pharmacy for their workplace problems, he noted.

Associations help shape the direction of our profession. In a recent white paper, the American Pharmaceutical Association, the National Association of Chain Drug Stores, and the National Community Pharmacists Association defined pharmacy as a profession that, in addition to being responsible for the safe dispensing of medications, is expanding to incorporate pharmaceutical care services. It's an example of how pharmacy associations work together to achieve goals on behalf of all pharmacists. Supporting state and national associations with your membership dollars helps promote pharmaceutical care and payment for patient care services. When you think of it, the cost is pretty reasonable. You probably pay a lot more per year for your cable television or cell phone service.

Strength in Numbers

Over the past 20 years or so, chiropractors and optometrists have been successful at creating a demand for their services and getting paid for them, probably as a result of their active involvement in associations that represent their interests. Optometrists used to dispense eye glasses. Now they have gained prescriptive authority in some states, and they co-manage patients with ophthalmologists, splitting a portion of follow-up fees after refractive surgery and cataract removal. The optometry profession should be a model for pharmacy to follow.

If higher numbers of pharmacists joined pharmacy associations and made the effort to voice concerns about workplace issues, we would be more likely to resolve them. Solutions will not come overnight, but there is strength in numbers. With greater membership, pharmacy associations would have greater support to expand professional responsibilities into such areas as basic screening services, monitoring patient outcomes, and collaborating with physicians about patients under their care.

 Idea #95 Become actively involved in your pharmacy organizations.

Contact your state or national association and ask if you can serve on a committee. Most likely there are several committees you can choose from, including Professional Affairs, Legislative Affairs, or Long Term Care. The time commitment may be as little as attending two or three meetings a year.

As you become more familiar with the association and its needs, you might consider serving in the house of delegates or running for a seat on the board of directors. Whatever level of commitment you decide to make, the first step—contacting the association—is essential. If you can't find time to serve the association directly, at least go to the meetings. The networking and educational opportunities are well worth the investment.

Idea #96 Attend at least one major meeting each year.

Among the professional meetings available to pharmacists are major annual conferences lasting up to five days and midyear educational sessions that take place over as few as one or two days. They cover just about anything you might need to know: disease management, pharmaceutical care, innovative software, using the Internet, automated prescription filling machines . . . you name it. Some state pharmacy groups also hold regional "town hall" meetings that last just a few hours and focus on one or two topics.

Equally important to your education is the forum that these meetings provide for pharmacists to collect and exchange ideas. It is a common meeting ground for networking with other pharmacists, learning new approaches, and sharing thoughts. I gathered many of the ideas in this book through conversations with other pharmacists at pharmacy meetings, as well as from educational sessions I attended. Pharmacy colleagues I've met at meetings have lifted me up when I was down on the profession. If you're reading this book because you need ideas to reduce stress or improve professionalism, you should know that there are many more where these came from. Simply make the effort to get out there and learn from others.

Idea #97 Teach inhaler technique at the consultation window.

If you're having difficulty deciding what to do with the extra time you have after making changes described earlier in this book, teaching patients the proper technique for using their inhalers is a good place to start. It's a skill that can be taught right at the consultation area—which might be a window or section of the pharmacy counter—and therefore doesn't require a separate, sit-down counseling space.

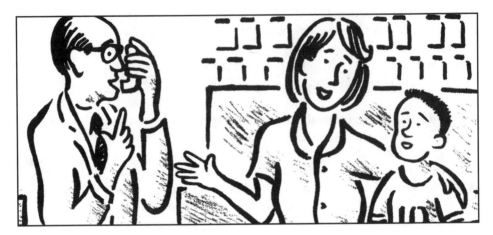

Teaching asthma patients inhaler technique shows that you care about their ability to benefit from their medication. It also demonstrates to them and the other people around you that you are a patient educator.

I recommend that all pharmacists talk with their pharmaceutical representatives who handle asthma products. Ask for a couple of placebo inhalers to use as demonstration devices. This is a simple and effective way to get more involved with educating patients.

When training patients to use proper inhaler technique, briefly describe the differences between a "rescue" inhaler and a "preventative" inhaler. This helps to keep them from discontinuing their preventative inhaler if they perceive no immediate benefit—a sort of prospective, rather than retrospective, intervention. The better patients understand how their medication works, the more likely they are to use it correctly.

Discussing asthma with patients may lead to other interventions, such as recommending a spacer or a peak flow meter, or teaching patients how to use a peak flow meter to optimal advantage. If you aren't comfortable with your asthma education skills, a one-day certificate course can help bring you up to speed.

At our pharmacy, we also have a six-inch plastic model of a trachea and bronchi that shows a normal, healthy bronchus, and an inflamed one. (It even comes with a disgusting-looking mucous plug.) It's great for convincing both kids and adults to use their maintenance medications regularly.

Keep in mind that doing training at the consultation window can be a little uncomfortable at first. It's far from private, and sometimes there can be quite an audience watching. But it's a simple, easy way to begin offering a patient care service, and allowing others to watch helps promote your skills and change patients' perceptions of you.

Idea #98 Ask yourself, "Is my job a perfect match for me?"

Do you work in a pharmacy environment that is professionally unrewarding for you? Do you feel overwhelmed on a daily basis? Are you getting the opportunity to put your professional skills to use? If the answers to these questions are not what you think they should be, then maybe it's time to consider a new work environment.

The pharmacist job market is booming right now. Pharmacists are receiving benefits packages that include free automobile leases, tuition reimbursement, extra vacation, stock options, and a hefty sign-on bonus to boot. If there was ever a good time to be a "free agent," it's now. If you have a pharmacy license, you can pick and choose where you want to work.

There is no panacea for the many problems we face, but the future of our profession and our personal wellness depend heavily on what we accept in our current work environments. As professionals, each individual pharmacist must start making decisions that will affect how pharmacy will be practiced in the future. If we do nothing and continue to work in jobs we don't like, we become obstacles to positive changes.

You might think, "What I do doesn't matter," or "How will what I do as one pharmacist change the outcome of our profession?" But we have to start somewhere. Pharmacists today are in a position to literally carve out what they want the profession to look like.

One pharmacist I know moved to the east coast when her husband was relocated. When she discovered how unprofessional the work environment was at her new job, she immediately made the decision to seek employment elsewhere. She was worried that because the pharmacy didn't follow laws about patient consultation and other matters, she risked losing her pharmacy license. Two days after she quit, she received five offers for other positions, and accepted one with a family-run independent pharmacy. "It was a tremendous pay cut," she said—roughly a 10% drop—but she was happy to have found a professional environment she could feel comfortable working in.

Anthony Robbins, a nationally renowned speaker on personal success, says in his book *Unlimited Power*: "One of the keys to success is making a successful marriage between what you do and what you love." A couple of paragraphs later, Robbins talks about "workaholics" and how their jobs challenge and excite them. He recommends working your way toward jobs that are conducive to such enthusiasm. "If you can find creative ways to do your job, it will help you to move toward work that's even better. If you decide work is mere drudgery, just a way to bring home a paycheck, chances are it will never be anything more," Robbins says.

Pharmacists should see their job as a two-way street. When employers think pharmacists aren't fulfilling their responsibilities, they have the option of firing them. By the same token, if a pharmacist thinks an employer isn't fulfilling his or her need for a professional work environment, it's best to leave and find a job where the pharmacist's goals and employer's vision are better aligned. But before you take that step, discuss rational solutions with your supervisor in your current situation. If you feel that you are not making any progress, then it may be time to consider your options.

Before accepting a new position, it's a good idea to interview prospective employers carefully to help ensure the job is a good match for you. Be specific and ask:

- How many prescriptions are processed per day?

- How many people will I be working with daily?

- What does my employer think my primary responsibility is?

- Will I have other responsibilities? What are they?

- What is my prospective employer's vision for the future of pharmacy? Does the employer have an action plan for getting there?

- Why should I choose to work for your company rather than another? (If you don't get specific answers, ask probing questions about working conditions and the ability to counsel patients.)

Also, interview some current employees to see what their working conditions are like. Some sample questions:

- How long have you worked here?

- Have you worked anywhere else?

- What do you like about working here, and what do you dislike?

- Do you get ample time for breaks and lunch?

- Do you have time to counsel patients and work on solving their drug therapy problems?

- Do your company and your supervisor treat you like a health care professional? Or are they primarily concerned with cranking out prescriptions?

- Are you required to work overtime? If yes, do you get paid extra for it?

- Why should I choose to work for this company rather than another?

Typically, when an employer hires someone, the new employee is on probation for 90 days. Why shouldn't employees adopt the same strategy? If pharmacists took the attitude that they've placed their new employer on probation, they might be more comfortable leaving if the job didn't meet their expectations. Recent graduates: hold off on purchasing that new car until you know for sure that you plan to stay a while.

Some pharmacists are taking a lot of abuse, such as working in understaffed conditions, putting in 12-hour days, and not being able to take a lunch break. Conditions like these affect your personal well-being, your health, your job satisfaction, and your family. If your child enrolled in a school with a psychologically abusive environment, and nothing was being done to change it, would you find a more suitable school? Of course you would. Pharmacists who are unsatisfied with pumping out hundreds of prescriptions every day might consider working in a low-volume start-up, an independent pharmacy, a hospital, or a long-term care pharmacy with lower volume or better staffing. Contrary to what you might think, every employer and every work environment will be different. If you make a wrong decision, accept that you made a mistake and try again.

An option for pharmacists who are seeking someplace new is to work for a relief service for a while. These services—similar to temporary agencies for clerical personnel—give you a chance to test the waters by working for several different pharmacies. Eventually you get a feel for each pharmacy's culture, and you can decide where you are willing to fill in. If you really enjoyed working at a particular pharmacy, and they had an opening, perhaps they would buy you out of your contract with the relief agency.

When you seek a new position, try talking to several pharmacists within a 25- to 30-mile radius of your house. Ask if they are hiring and learn a little about their philosophy and work style. Give potential employers your resume and call them every two to three months to let them know you're still interested.

Steer Clear of Sweatshops

A friend of mine is a pharmacist at a low-volume supermarket pharmacy. He works some 12-hour days, but he never worries about taking breaks to go to the restroom and he often gets periods of 10 to 15 minutes in which no phones ring and no patients need attention. He always has plenty of time to sit down and eat. "When patients need my help I spend as much time as necessary with them," he said. "There are even times of boredom, but I have my sanity and a sense of dignity. I don't feel like I'm working in a sweatshop."

Idea #99 Fax "SOAP notes" to medical records.

To recent graduates and pharmacists who work in hospital or long-term care settings, "SOAP note" is a familiar term, but other pharmacists may not know that it refers to a patient documentation style used by doctors and nurses. Many pharmacists in community settings have started formulating SOAP notes in recent years. But even pharmacists who don't use SOAP notes themselves need to learn how to speak physicians' language if they want to help care for and manage patients. The initials stand for:

- Subjective patient information.
- Objective patient data.
- Assessment of this information.
- Plan, or your recommendation for care.

Subjective data is information that the patient tells you. It can be symptoms, social or medical history, how much the patient drinks, smokes, and exercises, or any information that cannot be directly observed or measured.

Objective data is signs that you observe, such as a rash, edema of the leg, gangrene, and so on. It is also information that you can measure, such as height, weight, temperature, blood pressure, respiratory rate, quality of respirations, pulse, blood glucose, and cholesterol.

Assessment is your interpretation of the subjective and objective data. By putting it all together, you form a professional opinion about what the data mean. You are not diagnosing the patient, you are simply making an assessment of the information. Pharmacists have been doing this for years, helping appraise patients' signs and symptoms so as to recommend the appropriate over-the-counter (OTC) product or refer the patient to a physician's care.

Plan is your course of action. What are you going to do or recommend for this patient? Will a certain OTC product be a logical choice for now, or should the patient see a physician immediately? Does the patient require more information or training? Should you discuss with the patient his reasons for not complying with a

Sample SOAP Note to a Physician

Professional Pharmacy
1278 Medical Circle
Madison, WI 53704

To Fax # 608-555-5555

Attention: Dr. Brandon Smith
From: Brenda L. Jacobs, RPh, CDE   Phone: 555-1212
Re: Patient John R. Doe   d.o.b. 4/9/82

Problem: Noncompliance with asthma therapy.

Subjective: Patient dislikes the taste that the steroid inhaler leaves in his mouth. Has difficulty sleeping through the night. Recently, he has not been able to mow the lawn without taking a break.

Objective: John has been doubling the use of his short-term beta-agonist inhaler. He appears to be using accessory muscles when breathing. Peak flow measurement has been about 50% of his maximum. Normal for John is about 80-85%. John is wheezing bilaterally.

Assessment: John's breathing has deteriorated, resulting in progression and lack of control of his asthma.

Plan: Re-evaluate medication regimen. Consider changing steroid inhaler to one he can tolerate, or add leukotriene inhibitor qHs. John and I discussed the importance of preventative treatment of his asthma. He has an appointment with you in two weeks, and has agreed to use his steroid inhaler until you can re-evaluate.

Professionally,

Brenda L. Jacobs, RPh, CDE

medication or care plan? Should you work with the patient to arrive at a more suitable care plan he can live with?

In the medical profession, a separate SOAP note is created for each health problem that a patient has. Before a SOAP note can be started, all the patient's problems must be identified and documented in the "problem" list. Then SOAP notes are generated.

Most pharmacists work with only one problem and SOAP note per patient. We fax our SOAP notes to the physician's office right after we meet with the patient. We've learned that if the patient has a potentially serious problem and the SOAP needs immediate attention, it is best to follow up with a phone call. When the SOAP is not urgent, it is best to fax the SOAP to the medical records department for placement in the patient's chart. This way the information is in the chart at the patient's next doctor visit, demonstrating that we communicated a specific problem to the doctor. We've discovered that if we fax a SOAP note directly to the physician, it most likely will not make it into the patient's record.

Learning Assessment Skills

I learned valuable patient assessment and care skills by volunteering for an ambulance service for 11 years. The training provided by local ambulance services is usually free of charge, and if you sign on as a volunteer you have a great opportunity to polish your skills under the guidance of an experienced mentor. Some state and national associations, colleges of pharmacy, nursing programs, and physician assistant curricula offer courses on patient assessment. You learn how to take vital signs, use a stethoscope, auscultate the lungs and heart, take blood pressure, check pupils and reflexes, do cognitive assessments, and document your findings. Even if you don't use all the skills immediately, having this background can help you better understand patient records. A small book of medical abbreviations is also a useful tool for pharmacists.

In most cases, let patients know that you will be communicating with their physician by fax. (A rare exception to informing patients of your actions might be when you are contacting the physician regarding concerns about narcotic overuse.) Explain that you want to give the doctor pertinent information that may improve the patient's level of care. If necessary, also fax over a copy of the patient's refill history so that the physician is aware of how well the patient complies with therapy and knows which medications other physicians are giving the patient.

Idea #100 Start using the HCFA-1500 form.

SEE
RELATED
IDEA
#39

To bill or not to bill . . . that is the question. If you decide to bill for your services, you have two choices. You can bill the patient, or you can bill the insurance company. Billing the patient means you get your payment up front, but if the patient objects to the amount you charge, your payment may not reflect the true value of your time and services. When you bill the insurance company you can submit whatever you have decided is the appropriate amount for your time and services—but you may not get paid at all, if pharmacists are not recognized in that state as "providers." And it's a hassle to generate bills and resubmit them when they are denied.

Either way, you must establish standard fees based on the amount of time you spend with the patient and the level of care provided. Most pharmacists have set the value of billable time at $90 to $120 an hour.

If you would like to bill the patient's insurance company, you will need to use a HCFA-1500 form—the same form that the Health Care Financing Administration established for Medicare billing. You need the following three things to bill using the HCFA-1500 form:

1. The patient's signature (or a signature on file at your pharmacy).

2. A diagnosis code (also known as an ICD-9 code, from the International Classification of Diseases). This must be obtained from the physician's office, so that you are not accused of diagnosing. Physicians are becoming accustomed to sharing this information for drug approvals, and will often give it to you if you say that you need it to send in the bill for a patient.

3. A CPT (Common Procedural Terminology) code, which you assign according to the level of service you provide. The most common codes are 99201-5 and 99211-5. Discussing these codes in detail is beyond the scope of this book, but you can get further information at continuing education presentations or by talking with pharmacists who have gotten paid.

Some pharmacists send along a "Certificate of Medical Necessity" from the physician's office. This is a letter from the physician stating that the services provided by the pharmacist were necessary, and that the physician authorized them. The jury is still out on whether this helps or hinders receiving payment. Some pharmacists prefer not to send these, for fear that they will become a standard requirement for every patient care activity we handle.

It may be helpful to send along with the HCFA-1500 form a description of the service you provided and how it benefited the patient. You can use the following patient care documentation form. Experiment with sending it into the insurance company or saving it as documentation of the service provided and proof of the "signature on file" statement you make on the HCFA-1500 form.

Be sure to obtain permission from patients to bill their insurance companies. Always bill their major medical insurance provider, not their prescription drug insurance provider.

If you don't tell a patient up front that your consultation involves a fee, or you simply don't realize how much time you will be spending with the patient beforehand, you still have an opportunity to charge for your time. The patient may say, "How much do I owe you?" If so, consider saying something like this: "I'm glad you asked. Our standard fee for this service is $___. The service provided today, along with the time we spent together, should have a positive impact on your health. Some insurance companies have started to reimburse pharmacists for their professional services. If you would be kind enough to allow me to make a copy of your medical insurance card, and sign the form, I will charge you a $10 copay, and bill the remaining $___ to your insurance company." Or you could charge patients the entire fee, and let them submit it to their insurance company themselves.

Patient Care Documentation Form

Name _____d.o.b. _____

Address _____

Name of (referring) physician _____

DEA# _____ ICD-9 code_____

Service provided (box 19) _____

_____

Date of Service _____CPT code_____

Time spent_____Fee _____

Outcome:_____

_____

Estimated savings to the health care system: _____

_____

See attached copy of major medical card.

I, _____, received the above

services and authorize Pharmacy Consulting Services to bill for them.

Signed _____Date_____

Many pharmacists don't believe that patients will pay you to sit down and help them. They are surprised when a patient asks, "How much do I owe you?" Once I wrote an article on this subject entitled, "What Will You Say When They Ask?" I learned that a common response by pharmacists is, "Oh . . . nothing."

The next time you spend 10 minutes solving a patient's health or medication problem, and the patient asks your fee, say this if you do not have a standard fee established: "Thank you for asking. We're trying to justify to our company the benefits of helping people this way more frequently. To promote its value, we need to be reimbursed for our time. If you would like to pay the cashier a $10 contribution for this service today it would be greatly appreciated."

If you design a training program for patients with diabetes or offer other patient care services, you need to consider how much you will charge for them. Be confident in your ability and don't undervalue your services. Keep trying until you succeed in getting paid by the patient or insurance company. Consider offering something that no one else is offering, like computerized data management downloads from the patient's blood glucose monitor. You could provide this service for one year free of charge (included in your initial consultation fee of $30). Every time you discuss your programs with patients, you are communicating that you have information that will benefit them in a unique way.

Idea #101 Think win-win-win-win-win.

We've all heard it said that people should "think win-win." When it comes to pharmacy, however, I believe the expression should be: "Think win-win-win-win-win."

If we focus our mission on truly helping patients, <u>patients will win.</u> They will receive a higher quality of health care and, as a result, a better quality of life.

If patients win, it's reasonable to conclude that <u>physicians win</u> by managing patients' health more cost-effectively.

If the patient's health is managed more effectively, then <u>insurance companies win</u> by reducing costs. (The patient also shares in those savings through reduced premiums.)

If pharmacists use their professional skills to effectively manage patients' health, then it stands to reason that <u>pharmacists win,</u> too. When insurance companies see reduced costs and better patient outcomes, they will be more willing to reimburse pharmacists for their professional services. Ultimately, pharmacists will be able to spend more time on patient care and less time on technical functions.

<u>Pharmacy owners and employers win</u> because pharmacists who are reimbursed for professional services can delegate technical functions to others. Such functions can be handled by technicians at a lower cost to the company. More importantly, the owner or employer can

offer a valuable service that distinguishes their pharmacy from the competition.

Since implementing the strategies I have shared with you, our pharmacists have seen a positive change in our patients and in what they expect from us. We no longer skip lunch or delay restroom breaks. We work in a busy, yet professional, work environment. I hope you can put these ideas to work to improve your own work environment.

In his book, *The Seven Habits of Highly Effective People*, leadership trainer Stephen Covey advised, "Begin with the end in mind." It's a great approach. Many people who achieve their goals attribute their success to visualizing the outcome before they even get started, and then working backwards. Decide what you want your work environment to be like and how you want your professional future to unfold, and go for it.

We have a challenge and an opportunity to design our own future with better patient care in mind. Let us begin by taking the small steps necessary to make it happen.

A Model for the Future

Pharmacists are uniquely positioned to provide patient care services. I am both enthusiastic and optimistic about our future role. Eventually, I envision an arrangement with physicians similar to the one optometrists in our state have with ophthalmologists.

The optometrist in our building co-manages patients with area ophthalmologists. Written correspondence transmitted by fax machine keeps each provider informed about their patients' health status. A percentage of the surgical or exam fee goes to the optometrist for follow-up care, so the ophthalmologists can maximize their efficiency.

Pharmacists co-managing certain disease states with physicians in the same manner would go a long way toward creating a seamle   ntinuum of care.

SUGGESTED READING

For further reading on customer service, time management, pharmaceutical care, and professional success, check out these titles.

Blanchard K, Bowles S. *Raving Fans: A Revolutionary Approach to Customer Service.* New York, NY: Morrow; 1993.

Covey SR, Merrill AR, Merrill RR. *First Things First: To Live, to Love, to Learn, to Leave a Legacy.* New York, NY: Simon & Schuster; 1994.

Robbins A. *Awaken the Giant Within: How to Take Immediate Control of Your Mental, Emotional, Physical & Financial Destiny.* New York, NY: Simon & Schuster; 1991.

Robbins A. *Unlimited Power.* New York, NY: Fawcett; 1986.

Rovers JP, Currie JD, Hagel HP, et al. *A Practical Guide to Pharmaceutical Care.* Washington, DC: American Pharmaceutical Association; 1998.

INDEX

third party issues, 73, 94
diagnosis codes, 121–122, 152
director questions, 58–59
discount cards
    third party, 75–77
dispense as written (DAW)
    prescriptions, 99–100
dispensing errors
    avoiding, 88–89
doctors, 116–124
    collaboration with pharmacists,
    120–121, 124, 130, 156
    communicating with, 122–123
    direct phone numbers for, 124
    faxing SOAP notes to, 149–152
    order information standards
    for, 117
    refill authorizations from,
    32–33, 66–73
    requests for pharmacist to call,
    118–119
    telephone contact with, 104, 123
double checking
    by pharmacists, 88–89
double count, 26
drug ordering
    by technicians, 74
"drug police," 27

E
emergency medical technician
(EMT), 121
emotional distance, 28
employee roles, 32–33
exit statements, 59
expired prescriptions, 18–19, 69–71

F
fast service, 10
fax machine

prescription request to doctor
using, 119
refill procedure using, 67
sending SOAP notes to medical
records via, 149–152
training doctors/nurses to
use, 116
features
    defining, 134–136
fees
    collecting, 152–155
    estimating, 63
    explaining, 134–136
filing tips, 45
first party charges
    elimination of, 46–47
forms. *See also* canned responses
    HCFA-1500 (Health Care Finance
    Administration), 152–155
    OTC consultation, 59–61
    patient care documentation, 154

G
golden triangle workspace, 86–87

H
HCFA-1500 form (Health Care
Finance Administration), 152–155
health care professional
    emphasis on, 54–55
Heckman, H. Edward, 99–100
hours
    cash register, 109–100
    technicians, 52–54
humor
    use of, 29–30

I
in-box
    management of, 44–46

inhaler technique
    teaching of
        at consultation window,
        143–145
insurance company. *See also* third
party issues
    billing of, 152–155
    communicating with, 95–97
    vacation supplies, 74–75
intake time, 82–83
intake window
    promoting call ahead refill
    service at, 17
intervention
    versus override, 20
interviewing
    with prospective employers,
    146–147

J
job changes
    preparing for, 146–147
job market, 145
job satisfaction, 145–148

L
license
    posting of, 140
local pharmacy meetings, 143
    doctors at, 120–121, 124, 130
    technicians at, 35–36

M
magnetic tracking systems, 112–113
mailboxes
    for technicians/staff, 33–34
mail-out prescriptions
    payment policy for, 46–47
managers
    tips for, 44–55

marketing, 140
medical records
    faxing SOAP notes to, 149–152
meeting on paper (MOP)
    weekly, 51–52
miscounts
    patients' claims of, 27
mission statement
    creating, 40–41

N
National Association of Chain Drug
Stores, 141
National Community Pharmacists
Association, 141
National Drug Code (NDC) codes,
88–89
negative information
    conveying, 18–19, 24–25, 27–29
new patient information
    direct entry of, 37
newsletter
    pharmacist-physician, 130
nurses, 116–124
    communicating with, 122–123
    direct phone numbers for, 124
    order information standards
    for, 117

O
objective data, 149
Occupational Safety and Health
Administration (OSHA), 50–51
Omnibus Budget Reconciliation Act
of 1990 (OBRA '90), 61
optometry, 142, 156
ordering drugs, 74
OTC consultation form, 59–61
OTC section
    long-winded patients in, 59

override
    versus intervention, 20

P

patient(s)
    billing of, 152
    versus customer, 21
    delegating insurance issues to,
    73–74, 94, 96
    long-winded
        redirecting, 58–59
    needy
        speedy prescription filling
        for, 10
    offering your business cards to,
    138–139
    and refill expirations, 18–19,
    69–70
    responsibilities of, 8
    training of
        for call ahead refill service,
        14–18, 69–71
        to call doctors for refills,
        32–33, 66–73
patient assessment, 149
patient care
    versus customer service, 54
    pharmacist-technician
    collaboration in, 36
patient care area
    establishment of, 137
patient care documentation form, 154
patient consultation. *See* counseling
sessions
patient education
    about third party issues, 92–93
    at consultation window, 143–145
    funding for
        from pharmaceutical
        representatives, 130–131, 144

patient information
    direct entry of, 37
    standards for
        for doctors/nurses, 117
    verification of, 84
patient purchases
    register for, 108–109
patient questions
    telephone, 102–103
patient's name
    obtaining, 38–39
patient's phone number
    obtaining, 39
payment policies
    for mail-out prescriptions, 46–47
pharmaceutical care work environment, 88, 137
pharmaceutical representatives, 126–132
    appointment-only policy for,
    129–130
    drop-in visits by, 128–129
    funding from, 130–132, 144
    location of consultation with,
    127–128
    offering your business cards to,
    138–139
    time limit for, 126–127
pharmacist check station, 86–87
pharmacists
    collaboration with doctors,
    120–121, 124, 130, 156
    contact information, 138–139
    double checking of prescriptions
    by, 88–89
    functions of, 86
    future prospects for, 145
    interaction with doctors/nurses,
    122–123
    job satisfaction, 145–148
Pharmacy Audit Assistance Service

refill service
terminology
    for patient communication, 20
theft, 112
third party audit
    reducing risk of, 99–100
third party brochure
    designing, 92–93
third party discount cards, 75–77,
96–98
    cash in lieu of, 99
third party issues, 92–100. *See also*
insurance company
    dealing with, 25, 27
    delegating to patient, 73–74
    diagnosis codes, 121–122
    patient advocacy, 95–96
    patient education about, 92–93
third party rejection
    communicating, 93–95
    refill too soon, 117
"to do" box, 46
touch tone refill system, 16, 105–106
tracking systems
    prescription, 112–113
TRAF method, 44–45

V
vacation supplies
    handling, 74–75
value
    focus on, 7–8
visual cues, 24, 28–29
voice mail
    training doctors/nurses to
    use, 116
voice response system (IVR)
interactive
    for refills, 16, 105–106

W
wait
    apologizing for, 17
weekly meeting on paper (MOP),
51–52
work day
    taking control of, 58–64
work environment
    appearance of, 80–81
    perfect
        imagining, 8–9
    pharmaceutical care, 88, 137
workflow, 80–89
workspace
    golden triangle, 86